ACUTE PHASE OF ISCHEMIC HEART DISEASE AND MYOCARDIAL INFARCTION

DEVELOPMENTS IN CARDIOVASCULAR MEDICINE

VOLUME 21

series ISBN 90-247-2336-1

ACUTE PHASE
OF
ISCHEMIC HEART DISEASE
AND
MYOCARDIAL INFARCTION

edited by

A.A. JENNIFER ADGEY

Regional Medical Cardiology Centre
Royal Victoria Hospital
Belfast, N. Ireland

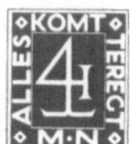

MARTINUS NIJHOFF PUBLISHERS
THE HAGUE / BOSTON / LONDON

Distributors:

for the United States and Canada
Kluwer Boston, Inc.
190 Old Derby Street
Hingham, MA 02043
USA

for all other countries
Kluwer Academic Publishers Group
Distribution Center
P.O. Box 322
3300 AH Dordrecht
The Netherlands

Library of Congress Cataloging in Publication Data   CIP
Main entry under title:

Acute phase of ischemic heart disease and myocardial infarction.

   (Developments in cardiovascular medicine ; v. 21)
   Includes index.
   Contents: Sudden death, ventricular fibrillation, ventricular defibrillation / A.A. Jennifer Adgey – A
new look at cardiopulmonary resusciation / Steven Ung, James T. Niemann, and J. Michael Criley –
Etiology of ventricular arrhythmias in the early phase of myocardial ischemia / Michiel J. Janse – [etc.]
   1. Coronary heart disease – Treatment.   2. Heart – Infarction – Treatment.   3. Ventricular fibrilla-
tion – Treatment.   4. Electric countershock.   5. Medical emergencies.   I. Adgey, A.A. Jennifer.
II. Series.
[DNLM: 1. Coronary disease. 2. Myocardial infarction. W1 DE997VME v. 21 / WG 300 A1896]
RC685.C6A29   616.1'23025   82-3628
ISBN 90-247-2675-1   AACR2

ISBN-13: 978-94-009-7581-1   e-ISBN-13: 978-94-009-7579-8
DOI: 10.1007/978-94-009-7579-8

What is all knowledge too but recorded experience, and a product of history; of which, therefore, reasoning and belief, no less than action and passion, are essential materials?

Thomas Carlyle (1795–1881)

CONTENTS

PREFACE

Although there are many books on ischemic heart disease and myocardial infarction, very few relate to the acute phase of the illness. Pre-hospital coronary care units have been operational for over a decade. In 1975 the first book detailing the operation and results of the out-of-hospital Belfast Mobile Coronary Care Unit was published (The Acute Coronary Attack – Pitman Medical). Nevertheless, deaths due to coronary artery disease still remain a major challenge in contemporary society. Sudden death is largely an out-of-hospital problem. Since ventricular fibrillation is an electrical accident and can be readily corrected when a limited area of the ventricle is depolarized, methods for its containment are essential.

The purpose of this book is to project the recent advances in the acute phase of ischemic heart disease. The early chapters document the history and recent developments in the understanding of ventricular fibrillation, ventricular defibrillation and cardiopulmonary resuscitation. The etiology of ventricular arrhythmias in the acute phase of myocardial ischemia in experimental animals is discussed with particular reference to the antiarrhythmic action of drugs. Factors observed in the initiation of ventricular fibrillation in patients outside the hospital are reviewed. The practical applications both in the field of biomedical engineering as applied to mobile coronary care and in the approach and impact of pre-hospital coronary care in the various communities in the United States of America, Canada, United Kingdom, and other countries in Europe are presented. The clinical profile and detailed pathology of victims of out-of-hospital ventricular fibrillation are described. Prevention of recurrent ventricular fibrillation in those resuscitated from ventricular fibrillation in the absence of acute myocardial infarction is also recorded along with the indications and use of the implantable defibrillator.

Some material is repeated within the varying chapters but this has been done for the convenience of the reader. I offer my appreciation to all the authors whose expert contributions made this book possible. Finally, it remains for me to thank Martinus Nijhoff Publishers for their invaluable help in the production of this text.

A.A. Jennifer Adgey

CONTRIBUTORS

ADGEY, A.A. Jennifer, Regional Medical Cardiology Centre, Royal Victoria Hospital, Grosvenor Road, Belfast BT12 6BA, N. Ireland.

ANDERSON, John, Ulster Polytechnic, Jordanstown, N. Ireland (formerly Regional Medical Cardiology Centre, Royal Victoria Hospital, Belfast).

CHAMBERLAIN, Douglas A., Royal Sussex County Hospital, Brighton BN2 5BE, England.

CRAMPTON, Richard S., University of Virginia School of Medicine, Cardiology Division, Box 158, Charlottesville, VA 22908, U.S.A.

CRILEY, J. Michael, Division of Cardiology, Harbor-UCLA Medical Center, 1000 West Carson Street, Torrance, CA 90509, U.S.A.

EISENBERG, Mickey S., Department of Medicine, University of Washington and Project Restart, Smith Tower Room 508, 506 Second Avenue, Seattle, WA 98104, U.S.A.

HEARNE, Thomas, Emergency Medical Services Division, King County and Seattle, WA, U.S.A.

JANSE, Michiel J., Department of Cardiology and Clinical Physiology, University Hospital, Wilhelmina Gasthuis, Eerste Helmersstraat 104, 1054 EG Amsterdam, The Netherlands.

KELLER, Martin D., Department of Preventive Medicine, The College of Medicine, The Ohio State University Hospital, 466 West 10th Avenue, Columbus, OH 43210, U.S.A.

LEWIS, Richard P., Division of Cardiology, The College of Medicine, The Ohio State University Hospital, 466 West 10th Avenue, Columbus, OH 43210, U.S.A.

LIBERTHSON, Richard R., Cardiac Unit, Massachusetts General Hospital, Boston, MA 02114, U.S.A.

MIROWSKI, Michel, Sinai Hospital of Baltimore and The Johns Hopkins University School of Medicine, Baltimore, MD 21215, U.S.A.

MOWER, Morton M., Sinai Hospital of Baltimore and the Johns Hopkins University School of Medicine, Baltimore, MD 21215, U.S.A.

NAGEL, Eugene L., Department of Anesthesia, University of Florida College of Medicine, Gainsville, FL 32611, U.S.A.

NIEMANN, James T., Department of Emergency Medicine, Harbor-UCLA Medical Center, 1000 West Carson Street, Torrance, CA 90509, U.S.A.

REID, Philip R., Sinai Hospital of Baltimore and the Johns Hopkins University School of Medicine, Baltimore, MD 21215, U.S.A.

RUSKIN, Jeremy N., Cardiac Unit, Massachusetts General Hospital, Boston, MA 02114, U.S.A.

STANG, John M., Division of Cardiology, The College of Medicine, The Ohio State University Hospital, 653 Means Hall, 466 West 10th Avenue, Columbus, OH 43210, U.S.A.

STUDD, Clive, Royal Sussex County Hospital, Brighton BN2 5BE, England.

UNG, Steven, Division of Cardiology, Harbor-UCLA Medical Center, 1000 West Carson Street, Torrance, CA 90509, U.S.A.

WATKINS, Levi, Sinai Hospital of Baltimore and the Johns Hopkins University School of Medicine, Baltimore, MD 21215, U.S.A.

1. SUDDEN DEATH, VENTRICULAR FIBRILLATION, VENTRICULAR DEFIBRILLATION – HISTORICAL REVIEW AND RECENT ADVANCES

A.A. JENNIFER ADGEY

1. HISTORICAL REVIEW

1.1. Sudden death

For many centuries, sudden death unrelated to trauma has been recognised as a clinical entity. In the first century A.D. Pliny the Elder studied many citizens of Rome – physicians, senators, and businessmen – who had dropped dead. With no post-mortems, these deaths were usually attributed to 'an act of the gods'. Frequent records of sudden death were made throughout the Middle Ages and in the seventeenth and eighteenth centuries. In 1560 Lusitanus wrote: 'A reverend abbot from the Isle of Croma, one or two miles distant from Ragusa, when he was in good health and talking to several persons, said that he suddenly felt pain in his heart and with his hand moved rapidly toward the region of the heart, he fell, though slowly, to the earth and rapidly lost all his animal faculties. When called in I said he was dead. Not only was the pulse at the metacarpium and the temples missing, but even no motion upon the heart could be perceived. In order to satisfy the assistants I brought to the nostrils a burning candle whose flame did not move at all. Also a bright mirror was advanced near the mouth and nothing of respiratory contraction was seen on it. We then applied a glass vessel filled with water upon the thorax but the water was unmoved'. Lancisi [1] performed post-mortems on the citizens of Rome who died suddenly during 1705–1706, and found a natural cause for death in every case and he referred particularly to diseases of the blood vessels with 'obstruction therefrom of the free flow of blood'.

Sudden death due to coronary artery disease still remains one of the greatest challenges in contemporary society. It has been stated that coronary artery disease 'is extremely common and highly lethal, which frequently attacks without warning and in which the first symptoms are all too often the very last. Also, it is a disease which can be silent even in its most dangerous form' [2].

In 1966, there were 115 000 deaths from coronary heart disease in the United Kingdom. Each year in the United States approximately 800 000 individuals suffer an acute myocardial infarction, of whom approximately 550 000 die. More than half of the 550 000 deaths occur outside the hospital. Two-thirds of the deaths from coronary artery disease of those aged less than 65 years are unexpected and occur outside hospital [2]. More than one-half of the deaths are sudden and occur within

Adgey, AAJ (ed): Acute phase of ischemic heart disease and myocardial infarction.
© *1982, Martinus Nijhoff, The Hague, Boston, London. ISBN-13: 978-94-009-7581-1*

one hour of the onset of the first symptom. Two-thirds of sudden coronary deaths occur among patients who do not have previous clinical or electrocardiographic evidence of coronary artery disease. Death is more likely to be sudden in younger individuals and sudden coronary death is more likely in men than in women.

Sudden death and ventricular fibrillation are considered synonymous, since in more than 90% of sudden deaths outside hospital, ventricular fibrillation has been documented. Sudden death need not be a manifestation of an acute myocardial infarction but may represent a brief ischemic episode with a high tendency to recurrence [3]. Nevertheless, the long-term prognosis of patients with a clinically mild myocardial infarction complicated by early ventricular fibrillation is similar to that of patients whose coronary episode is not so complicated [4]. Thus a more optimistic outlook for the patient at risk of early sudden death complicating an acute myocardial infarction has been substantiated.

1.2. Ventricular fibrillation

Although ventricular fibrillation was probably known to Vesalius, it was Hoffa and Ludwig who, in 1850, provided the first clear description [5]. Their investigations showed that electrical stimulation of the mammalian heart led to ventricular fibrillation and death. Nevertheless, electrical currents to the heart using a direct current derived from a Leyden jar were first applied in the eighteenth century. In 1775 Abilgard [6] recorded that he 'shocked a single chicken into lifelessness and upon repeating the shock, the bird flew off and thus eluded further experimentation'. At approximately the same time Benjamin Franklin shocked goats and killed fowl with charges of static electricity. McWilliam in 1887 [7] suggested that sudden death was due to the development of ventricular fibrillation, and in 1889 [8] he indicated that there was a high probability of ventricular fibrillation being the cause of sudden death in patients with angina pectoris. Hoffman in 1911 [9] was the first to obtain an electrocardiogram showing ventricular fibrillation in the clinical situation, and in 1933, Hamilton and Robertson recorded ventricular fibrillation on the electrocardiogram of a patient during a fatal attack of angina pectoris [10]. The first reports of ventricular fibrillation as the cause of sudden death in man following acute myocardial infarction were made by Smith and Miller in 1939 [11, 12].

1.3. Cardio-pulmonary resuscitation

Tossach in 1743, resuscitating a coal miner overcome by gaseous fumes demonstrated the effectiveness of mouth to mouth respiration as a means of artificial ventilation [13]. The discovery by Kouwenhoven et al. [14] that it was possible to maintain adequate circulation by compression of the lower portion of the sternum removed the feeling of uselessness man had when confronted with a crisis in which a delay of four minutes was the limit for effective resuscitation [15].

3

1.4. Defibrillation

1.4.1. Internal
In 1899, Prevost and Battelli were able to defibrillate the ventricles of the dog's heart by applying either DC or AC countershocks directly to the myocardium [16]. Hooker et al. in 1933 [17] confirmed the work of Prevost and Battelli by their finding that internal cardiac massage and the direct application of AC shock to the ventricles corrected experimental ventricular fibrillation. In 1947, Beck et al. successfully corrected ventricular fibrillation in man by internal cardiac massage and direct application of AC countershock to the heart [18]. The patient was a 14-year-old boy undergoing thoracic surgery. Time had been shown to be a critical factor in determining clinical recovery from cardiac arrest. It had been stated in 1940 that if more than four minutes elapsed before resumption of an adequate cardiac output the chances for salvage without irreversible neurological damage were poor [19]. Widespread application of resuscitative measures was, therefore, limited.

The first hospital reports of successful resuscitation from ventricular fibrillation complicating acute myocardial infarction using internal cardiac massage and direct defibrillation appeared in 1956 [20, 21]. Yet in 1961 there had been less than twenty reports of patients successfully resuscitated [22, 23]. It was widely assumed that patients developing cardiac arrest in association with coronary artery disease had such severe disease that resuscitation would be unsuccessful despite the fact that many pathological studies had shown that the amount of myocardial damage was not infrequently small.

1.4.2. External
In 1809 Burns [24] stated: 'Where, however, the cessation of vital action is very complete, and continues long, we ought to inflate the lungs, and pass electric shocks through the chest: the practitioner ought never, if the death has been sudden, and the person not very far advanced in life, to despair of success, till he has unequivocal signs of real death'; moreover, several workers showed that experimental ventricular fibrillation could be removed by transthoracic countershock [17, 25–27]. In spite of this the clinical application was delayed until 1956. In that year Zoll et al. demonstrated the clinical feasibility of transthoracic defibrillation using AC shock [28]. Lown et al. in 1962 introduced DC shock (capacitor discharge) [29]. Thus, resuscitative measures were available that could be rapidly applied by trained medical and auxiliary staff in the correction of ventricular fibrillation.

At present there is no satisfactory means of identifying the patient at risk of sudden death. Furthermore, no fully effective and safe long-term antiarrhythmic agent is available. It is also uncertain whether the long-term prophylactic administration of any currently available antiarrhythmic agent will decrease the incidence of sudden death from coronary artery disease. In view of the difficulties of predicting sudden death no satisfactory alternative to immediate defibrillation is available.

Although it is admirable that 15 million Americans have now been trained in cardiopulmonary resuscitation, there exists an inverse relationship between the duration of cardiopulmonary resuscitation and survival. Resuscitation places additional burdens on the already damaged myocardium. When ventricular fibrillation occurs the myocardial fibres contract asynchronously and at a very rapid rate with increased oxygen consumption. Even the shortest intervals of interrupted coronary flow must increase the degree of ischemia and enlarge the area of injury. Further damage to the myocardium may occur with prolonged external cardiac massage.

The correction of ventricular fibrillation is clearly imperative as early as possible after its development. Occasionally this can be achieved by 'thump version'. Chemical defibrillation using Bretylium Tosylate has been described. However, defibrillation by DC shock is usually required. In 1966, Pantridge and Geddes were the first to demonstrate the successful correction of ventricular fibrillation outside hospital using a portable defibrillator [30, 31].

2. ENERGY LEVELS FOR DEFIBRILLATION

For ventricular defibrillation in the correction of ventricular fibrillation, the majority of studies advocate the maximum stored energy of the defibrillator, which is 400 Ws. From this stored energy most commercially available defibrillators deliver 270–330 Ws through a resistance of 50 Ω. It was originally thought that depolarization of every cell in the ventricles was necessary to terminate ventricular fibrillation. However, it has been shown that successful defibrillation occurs when a critical mass of myocardium is depolarized [32]. Nevertheless, it has been indicated that the maximal energy delivered from commercially available defibrillators is insufficient to defibrillate 35% or more of subjects weighing over 50 kg and ineffective in 60% of patients weighing 90 to 100 kg [33]. These claims are based on retrospective clinical data and on experimental studies. From these data an energy dose weight concept has been proposed for the correction of ventricular fibrillation. The dosage recommended was '4 to 6 joules per kg body weight' delivered energy [34].

2.1. Body weight

In Belfast, in 394 episodes of ventricular fibrillation among 214 patients, shocks of 100 Ws stored energy were successful in 81% of episodes of ventricular fibrillation [35]. A single shock of 100 Ws stored energy succeeded in 67%. Shocks of 200 Ws stored energy succeeded in 95%, and a single shock of 200 Ws was successful in 85%. Body weight was not related to the chance of successful defibrillation with 200 Ws stored energy nor was the length of time the patient was in ventricular fibrillation. Of the few patients in the Belfast study who failed to be defibrillated by low energy shocks there was not a single failure with 400 Ws stored. The maximum delivered energy was 330 Ws.

Table 1. Successful defibrillation of patients >100 kg

Authors	Year	No. patients	No. episodes	Weight (kg)	Shocks Ws Stored/Delivered
Curry and Quintana [39]	1970	1	1	108	1×300
Lappin [40]	1974	1	1	145	1×400 (S)
Tacker et al. [41]	1975	1	1	102.5	3×300 (D)
Campbell et al. [35]	1977	2	3	102	200 or 400 (S)
DeSilva and Lown [42]	1978	1	1	190.1	1×400 (S)
Gascho et al. [43]	1979	4	12	101–225	$\leqslant 400$ (S)
Total		10	19	101–225	$\leqslant 400$ (S)

Other workers have failed to find a relationship between body weight and energy required for defibrillation. Gascho et al. [36] studied 88 patients using a maximum energy of 400 Ws (stored), and showed no relationship between energy for defibrillation and body weight (maximum weight 225 kg). Kerber and Sarnat [37] studied 52 patients with ventricular fibrillation using energies ranging from 200 to 400 Ws (delivered). Body weight and heart weight were not related to the success of defibrillation. They showed that higher energy shocks were not more effective for defibrillation and suggested that higher energies might have had a deleterious effect on the myocardium.

2.1.1. Patients $\geqslant 100$ kg
It has been estimated that if a damped sine wave defibrillator is used to defibrillate patients weighing more than 100 kg, a delivered energy in excess of 500 Ws would be necessary [38]. This has not been the experience of other workers. A review of the available literature has shown that of 19 episodes in 10 patients weighing 101–225 kg, energies of 400 Ws stored or less successfully corrected ventricular fibrillation (Table 1) [39–41, 35, 42, 43]. Collins et al. [44] Kerber and Sarnat [37] and Anderson and Suelzer [45] found that in 9 out of 14 patients (64%) weighing 100 kg or more, ventricular fibrillation was successfully corrected using a maximum delivered energy of 400 Ws or less (Table 2).

Table 2. Defibrillation of patients $\geqslant 100$ kg

Authors	Year	No. patients	Successful Defib.	Weight kg	Shocks Ws Stored/Delivered
Collins et al. [44]	1978	2	0	>100	400 (S)
Kerber and Sarnat [37]	1979	2	1	110, 159	200–400 (D)
Anderson and Suelzer [45]	1976	10	8	100–140	250

6

Table 3. No significant relationship between energy for defibrillation and heart weight

Authors	Year	No. patients	Etiology	Heart weight (g)	Energy Direct/Indirect Ws
Tacker et al. [46]	1978	100	Cardiac surgery	250–1,000*	1–30 (D)
Rubio and Farrell [47]	1979	30	Cardiac surgery	—	≤ 10 (D)
Kerber and Sarnat [37]	1979	22	—	320–750	200–400 (I)

* estimated

2.2. Heart weight

Tacker et al. failed to show a relationship between the energy required to correct ventricular fibrillation during open heart surgery and the weight of the heart estimated by the surgeon or at autopsy [46] (Table 3). Rubio and Farrell [47] made similar observations among 30 patients undergoing open heart surgery. Kerber and Sarnat [37] studied 22 patients who died following attempted defibrillation by

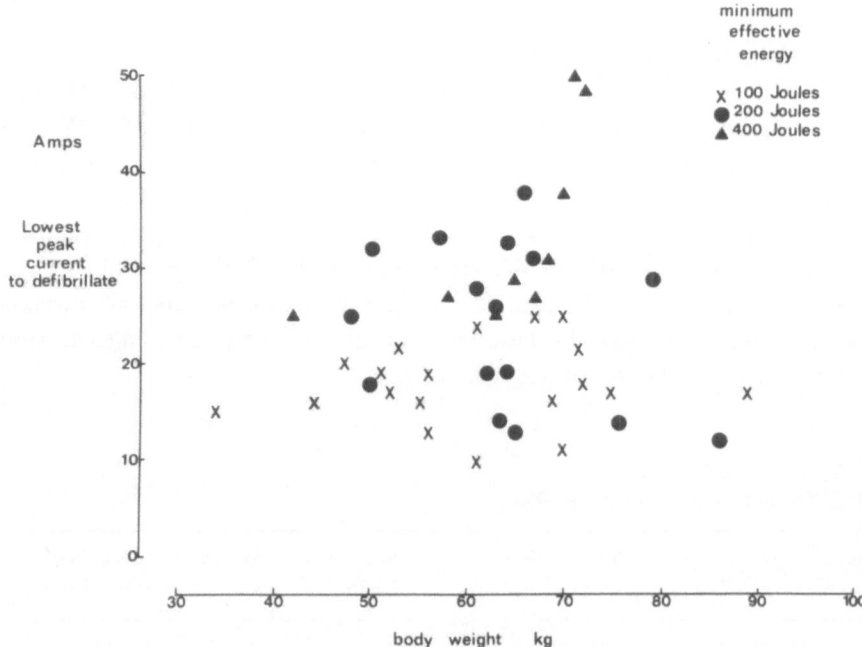

Figure 1. Lowest peak current for defibrillation and body weight in kilograms in the 44 patients. Minimum effective energy 100, 200, 400 J. Reproduced with permission [49].

7

2

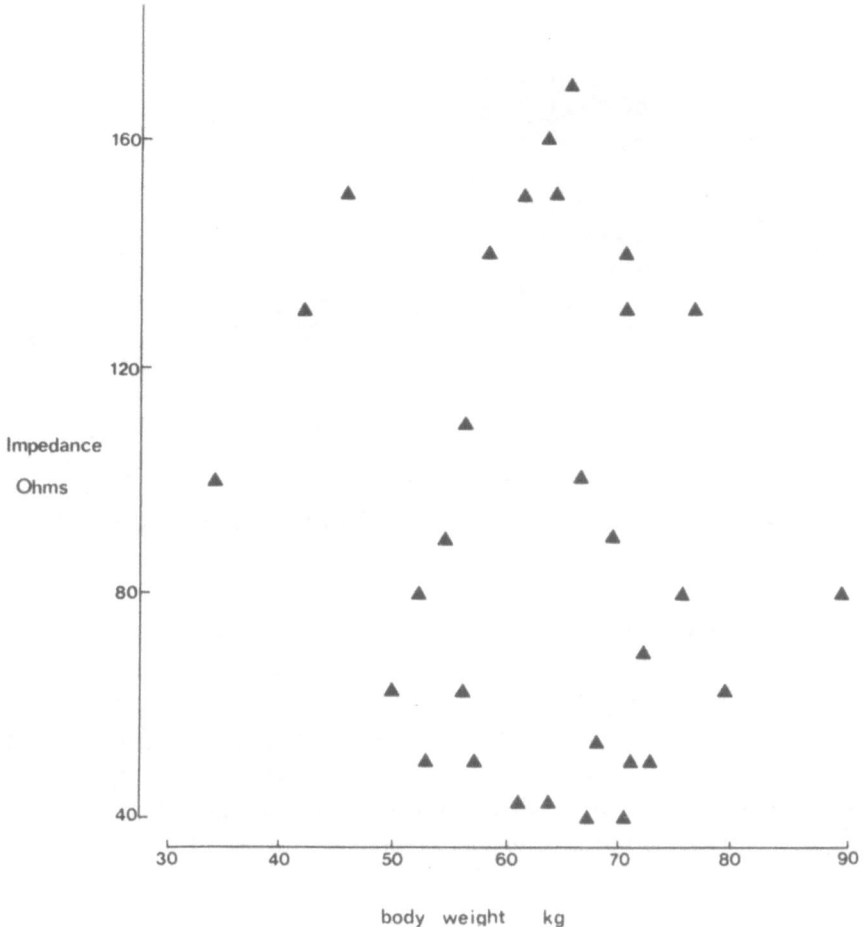

Figure 2. Transthoracic impedance plotted against body weight in kilograms in 31 patients. Reproduced with permission [49].

shocks of 200–400 Ws (delivered energy) applied to the chest wall. Heart weights ranged from 320 to 750 g. They found no relationship between heart weight and the energy required for defibrillation.

2.3. *Peak current and transthoracic resistance*

It has been postulated that peak current and, in particular, peak current per kg of body weight might be a better measure of the requirements for clinical ventricular defibrillation than delivered energy [48]. It has been considered that peak current for successful defibrillation might have a linear relationship to body weight, and that in adults 1 A per kg might be the current required for defibrillation [48]. The peak current required for defibrillation was measured in 44 patients who weighed

8

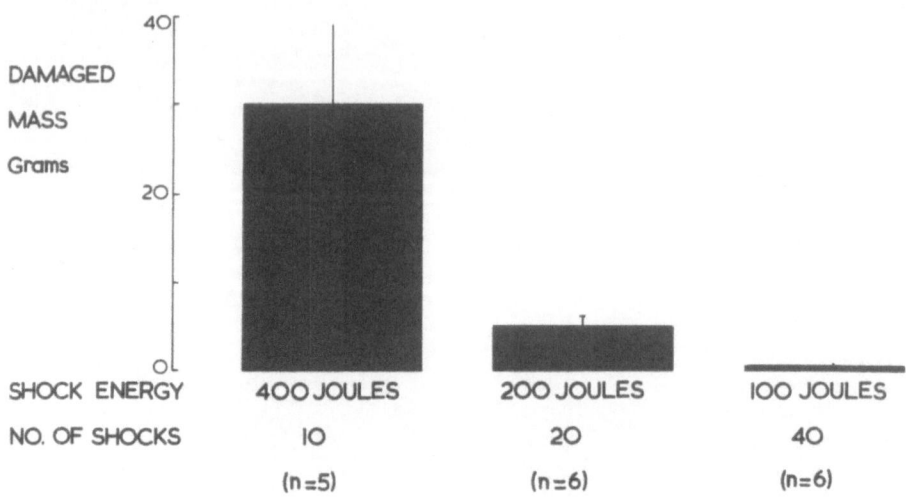

Figure 3. Amount of myocardial damage in g after DC countershocks (mean and $\pm$ SEM).

35–89 kg [49]. It varied from 0.14 to 0.71 A per kg (mean $0.37 \pm$ SEM 0.02 A per kg) (Figure 1). Thus, the average current required for defibrillation of adult patients is about one-third of that predicted from animal experiments. The transthoracic resistance was usually greater than $50\,\Omega$ and ranged from 40 to $170\,\Omega$ (mean $88 \pm 8.3\,\Omega$) (Figure 2). There was no relationship between the body weight and either the defibrillating current or the transthoracic resistance (Figures 1 and 2). Peak current per kg is not a better determinant of success of defibrillation than energy.

2.4. Myocardial damage

It has been argued that when the initial shock is of low energy it may have to be repeated, and that two low-energy shocks may cause more damage than a single shock of identical total energy. The effects of DC shock on the myocardium were investigated in 17 greyhound dogs weighing 21–37.5 kg (Figure 3) [50]. Eight-centimetre paddles were used and shocks synchronized to the R wave of the electrocardiogram were passed through the closed chest at 30-second intervals. The dogs were randomly allocated to three groups; group 1 received 10 shocks of 400 J, group 2 20 shocks of 200 J and group 3 40 shocks of 100 J. Three days later the animals were sacrificed and the beating hearts excised. The macroscopically damaged areas were then dissected and weighed. The damaged areas in group 1 weighed from 6.1 to 57.0 g (mean $30.1 \pm$ SEM 10.6 g), in group 2 from 0.5 to 9.4 g (mean $5.1 \pm$ SEM 1.3 g) and in group 3 from 0.1 to 2.1 g (mean $0.5 \pm$ SEM 0.3 g) (Figure 3). When the myocardial damage in groups 2 and 3 was compared with that in group 1, the differences were statistically significant ($P < 0.05$). These data do not suggest that low energy shocks will cause more myocardial damage than a single shock of identical total energy.

2.5. Successful defibrillation

It has been suggested that the use of energies of less than 300 Ws (delivered) will unnecessarily delay success in the correction of ventricular fibrillation. Since to ensure successful defibrillation it had been thought that the maximum stored energy of the defibrillator, i.e. 400 Ws, should be used for the initial shock, a recent study reported by Weaver et al. is of interest [51]. In a prospective randomized out-of-hospital trial they found that there was no difference in the success rate in the correction of ventricular fibrillation when patients received two 200 Ws stored (175 Ws delivered) shocks or two 400 Ws stored (320 Ws delivered) shocks. In both groups of patients an identical percentage of patients were resuscitated and survived to leave hospital. Furthermore, they go on to suggest that high energy shocks, i.e. 400 Ws stored, may cause significantly more cardiac toxicity as measured by a greater incidence of high degree atrioventricular block after correction of ventricular fibrillation. In addition, when one looks at the charge time for defibrillators (knowing the success rate with 100 and 200 Ws stored energy shocks), valuable seconds would be wasted as defibrillators are charged to 400 Ws stored (Table 4).

Since defibrillation with the least energy minimises the risk of myocardial damage, the lowest possible energy levels that effectively defibrillate should be used. From current clinical experience 400 Ws stored energy is in excess of that required for defibrillation in the majority of adult patients. It is suggested that the first shock is of 200 Ws stored energy. If this is unsuccessful, the 200 Ws shock should be repeated. If both are unsuccessful then 400 Ws stored energy should be used.

For the successful correction of ventricular fibrillation particular attention must be paid to paddle placement. One paddle is placed immediately to the right of the sternum and under the right clavicle and the other on the anterior axillary line in the fifth left intercostal space. The paddles are covered by a saline electrode-jelly to obtain maximum reduction in transthoracic impedance. Both paddles are firmly held on the chest wall. If paddles are placed in an incorrect position as shown

Table 4. Defibrillators

Stored energy Ws	Charge time (secs)			
	Pantridge portable	American optical 2015	Lifepak 33	Lifepak 5
100	2	2	6	3
200	4	4	10	6
400	8	7	21	10

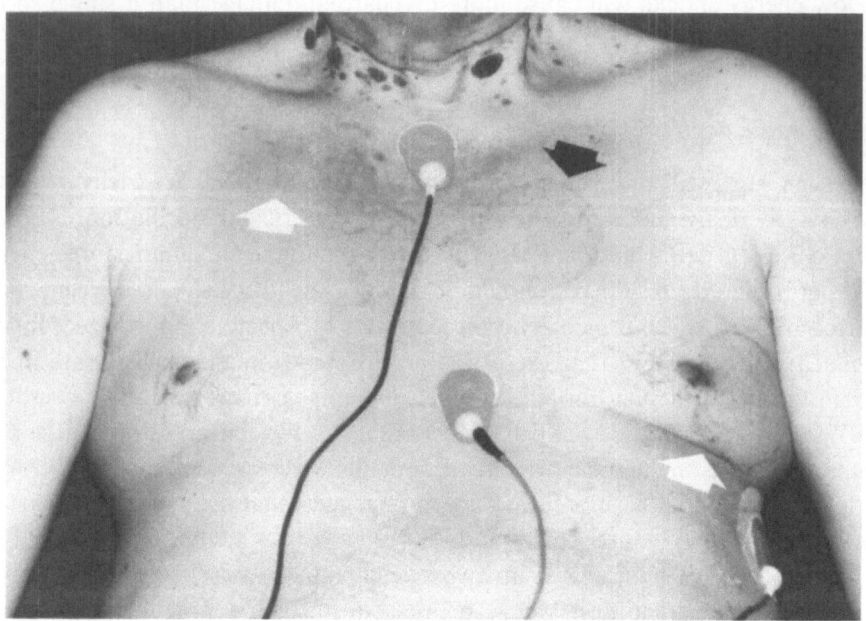

Figure 4. Erythematous rings following transthoracic defibrillation.
Black arrow — incorrect paddle position.
White arrows — correct paddle positions.

(Figure 4), then unsuccessful defibrillation is very likely to result.

The widespread availability of small inexpensive defibrillators is to be encouraged. Indeed, it might be desirable to have in certain factories and office blocks a defibrillator mounted beside the fire extinguisher.

3. THE INITIAL ARREST, VENTRICULAR FIBRILLATION – NUMBER OF SHOCKS

The number of DC shocks required to correct ventricular fibrillation during the initial arrest was previously unknown. Nonetheless, in the future development of defibrillators, particularly with reference to miniaturisation, it is helpful to ascertain the number of DC shocks used during this arrest.

The assessment was made in a retrospective study of 270 consecutive patients with ventricular fibrillation who were managed during the years 1973 and 1974 [52]. Of 141 patients who survived the initial episode, ventricular fibrillation complicated either an acute myocardial infarction or an acute ischemic episode. An arrest consisted of one or more episodes of ventricular fibrillation. The initial episode in 110 patients was primary ventricular fibrillation, i.e. ventricular fibrillation in the absence of cardiogenic shock or pump failure (Figure 5). Seventy-three of these had ventricular fibrillation within the first 12 h of the onset of symptoms. Fifteen

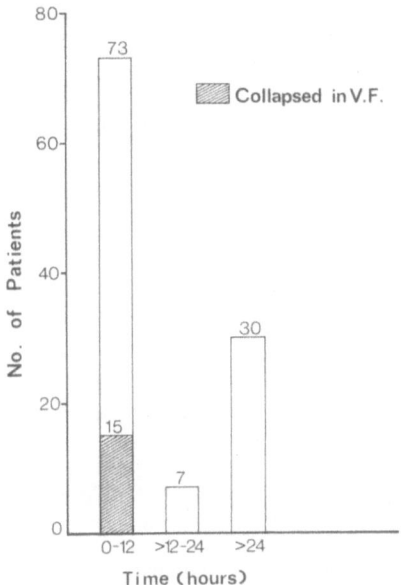

Figure 5. Interval between onset of symptoms and initial primary ventricular fibrillation in 110 patients with an acute myocardial infarction or an acute ischemic episode. Reproduced with permission [52].

collapsed in ventricular fibrillation.

At the initial arrest in these 73 patients, the number of DC shocks (200, 400 Ws stored) required to correct ventricular fibrillation ranged from 1 to 12 (mean 2) (Figure 6). Only 3 patients had 10 or more shocks. In 2 patients ventricular fibrilla-

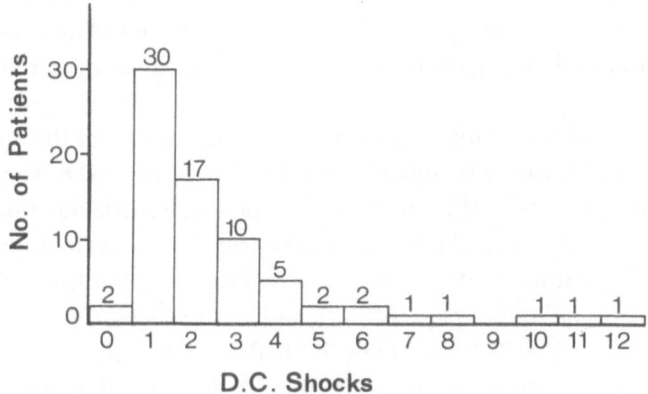

Figure 6. The number of shocks during the initial arrest in 73 patients with primary ventricular fibrillation within 12 h of the onset of symptoms. 0 − 'Thump-version' (2 patients). Reproduced with permission [52].

12

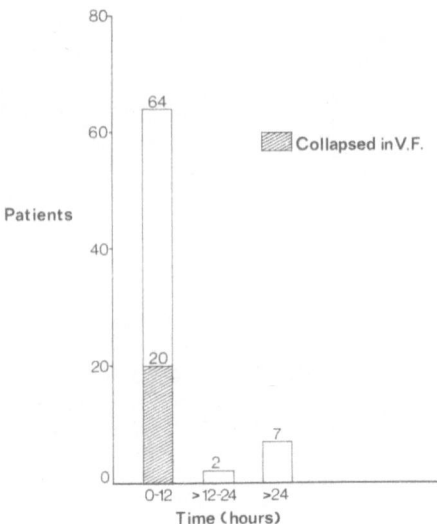

Figure 7. Interval from onset of symptoms to initial primary ventricular fibrillation in 73 patients with acute myocardial infarction. Reproduced with permission [53].

tion was successfully corrected by 'thump version.' Thirty-six of the 73 patients had a single arrest with a single episode of ventricular fibrillation. Twenty-six patients had a single arrest with 2 to 10 (mean 3) episodes of ventricular fibrillation. Eleven patients had several arrests. They varied from 2 to 3 arrests (mean 2) with 2 to 7 episodes (mean 2) of ventricular fibrillation for each arrest.

3.1. First hour of acute myocardial infarction

In a further analysis of 73 consecutive patients who were seen within one hour of an acute myocardial infarction and who survived the initial episode of primary ventricular fibrillation during the years 1972 to 1974, it was found that in 64 of them the initial arrest occurred during the first 12 hours from the onset of symptoms (Figure 7) [53].

For the successful correction of ventricular fibrillation during the initial arrest in these 73 patients, 27 patients required a single DC shock, 14 two DC shocks and only 2 required multiple shocks (Figure 8). In one patient ventricular fibrillation was corrected by 'thump version.' At this arrest, 35 of the 73 patients had a single episode of ventricular fibrillation, 14 had 2 episodes, and only 2 had multiple episodes. Thus in the initial arrest in these 73 patients, 67% had ≤2 episodes of ventricular fibrillation and 57% required ≤2 shocks. Only 7% had >10 shocks.

Ventricular fibrillation occurred within the first hour in 39 of these 73 patients. During this initial arrest, 16 patients required ≤ 2 DC shocks to correct ventricular fibrillation and only 3 patients required >10 shocks (Figure 9). An average of 2 shocks was required for each episode of ventricular fibrillation. At this early arrest

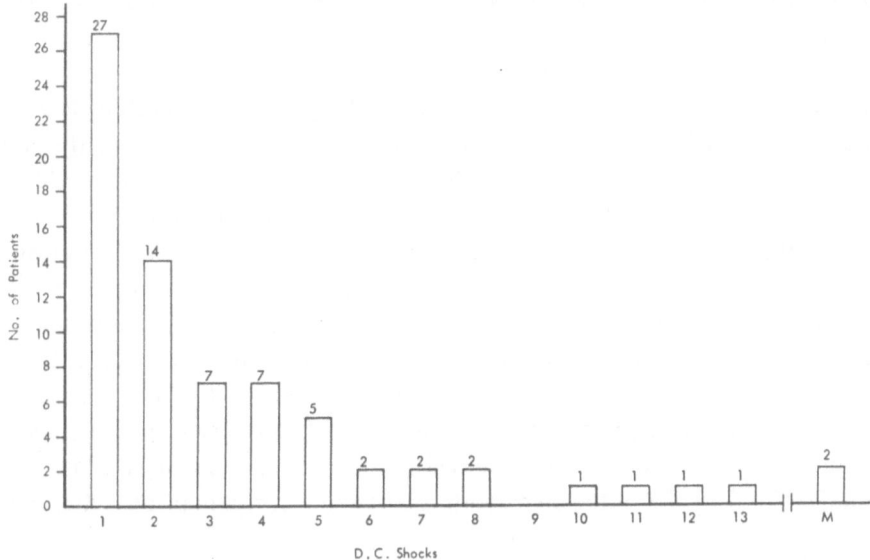

Figure 8. Number of DC shocks in the initial arrest (72 patients). In one patient ventricular fibrillation was corrected by 'thump-version'. M = Multiple >13 shocks. Reproduced with permission [53].

21 patients had a single episode, 10 had 2 episodes and only 2 had 5 episodes. Thus at the initial arrest in these 39 patients with ventricular fibrillation within the first hour, 80% had ≤2 episodes of ventricular fibrillation and 41% required ≤2 shocks to correct ventricular fibrillation. Only 8% required >10 shocks to terminate ventricular fibrillation.

3.2. Number of shocks

From these two studies [52, 53] it can be seen that a defibrillator capable of producing 8 DC shocks with a maximum stored energy of 400 Ws would have successfully defibrillated 90% and more of patients during the initial arrest.

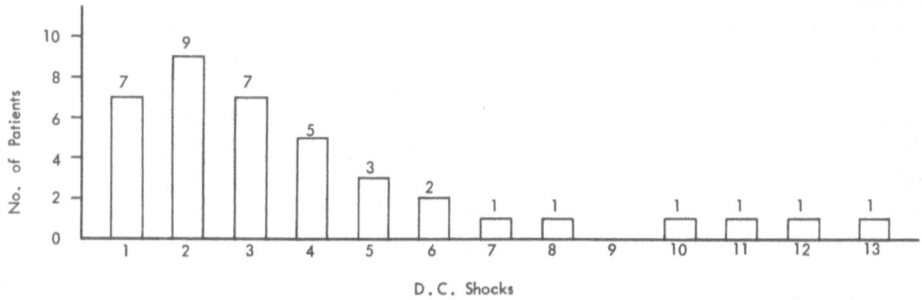

Figure 9. Number of DC shocks in the initial arrest within the first hour of acute myocardial infarction (39 patients). Reproduced with permission [53].

4. RECURRENCE OF VENTRICULAR FIBRILLATION IN ACUTE ISCHEMIC
   HEART DISEASE

Whilst ventricular fibrillation has been successfully corrected both outside and inside the hospital, little information is available on its recurrence during the period of hospitalisation. Lie et al. reported that of 400 consecutive patients with acute myocardial infarction, 18 developed primary ventricular fibrillation in hospital [54]. Twelve of the 18 patients had recurrent attacks of ventricular fibrillation during the period of hospitalisation. Lie and Durrer reported a total experience of 30 patients with primary ventricular fibrillation complicating acute myocardial infarction [55]. Eight of the 30 patients (27%) had recurrent attacks of primary ventricular fibrillation during hospitalisation. These were refractory to antiarrhythmic intervention and to cardiac pacing: El-Sherif et al. reported that, of 450 consecutive patients with acute myocardial infarction, 20 developed primary ventricular fibrillation during hospitalisation [56]. Six of the 20 patients (30%) had recurrent episodes during this period.

In a retrospective study [52] it was shown that, of 150 survivors of ventricular fibrillation out of 270 consecutive patients managed during the years 1973 and 1974, the initial episode of ventricular fibrillation in 141 patients complicated either an acute myocardial infarction (121 patients) or an acute ischemic episode (20 patients). The initial episode in 110 patients was primary ventricular fibrillation and in 31 patients it was secondary ventricular fibrillation. Recurrent ventricular fibrillation was defined as the recurrence of this dysrhythmia half an hour or more after its correction and restoration of a satisfactory circulation. No patient had a further immediate infarction, either prior to the initial episode or at the time of recurrence of ventricular fibrillation. Two patients had further pain approximately 1 h before the recurrence of ventricular fibrillation but there was no electrocardiographic evidence of further infarction. The period of hospitalisation ranged from 1 to 73 days (mean 23 days). Ninety-one patients survived hospitalisation.

Table 5. Recurrence of ventricular fibrillation in patients with acute myocardial infarction or an acute ischemic episode

	Patients	RVF
Total	141	41 (29%)
MI	121	31 (26%)*
AIE	20	10 (50%)*

* P < 0.05
RVF = Recurrence of ventricular fibrillation
MI = Myocardial Infarction
AIE = Acute ischemic episode
Reproduced with permission [52].

Table 6. Recurrence of ventricular fibrillation, primary and secondary ventricular fibrillation complicating acute myocardial infarction or an acute ischemic episode

VF	Patients MI		Patients AIE	
	Total	RVF	Total	RVF
Primary	94	19 (20%)*	16	8 (50%)
Secondary	27	12 (44%)*	4	2 (50%)

* P <0.05
Reproduced with permission [52].

4.1. Acute ischemia and acute myocardial infarction

Of the 141 patients, 41 (29%) had recurrent ventricular fibrillation during hospitalisation (Table 5). The incidence of recurrent ventricular fibrillation among those with an acute ischemic episode was almost twice that of patients who had had an acute myocardial infarction (Table 5). When patients are resuscitated from ventricular fibrillation outside hospital and discharged home, the incidence of recurrent out-of-hospital ventricular fibrillation is significantly greater when the initial episode of ventricular fibrillation complicates ischemic heart disease rather than acute myocardial infarction [57, 58]. This increased risk of recurrence among those with an acute ischemic episode may reflect continuing myocardial electrical instability. Haynes et al. [59] compared the 12 lead electrocardiograms of survivors from out-of-hospital ventricular fibrillation complicating ischemic heart disease with those of patients who were ambulatory and had had a myocardial infarction without ventricular fibrillation. They found that survivors of out-of-hospital ventricular fibrillation had a higher incidence of ventricular ectopics, greater prevalence of ST segment depression, T wave flattening and QTc prolongation. These differences between the two groups were independent of drug therapy.

4.2. Secondary ventricular fibrillation

When ventricular fibrillation complicates hypotension or heart failure it is likely to be recurrent. Of the 94 patients in this study with primary ventricular fibrillation complicating an acute myocardial infarction, 19 (20%) had recurrent ventricular fibrillation, whereas of the 27 patients with secondary ventricular fibrillation, 12 (44%) had recurrent ventricular fibrillation (Table 6). Thus the incidence of recurrence of ventricular fibrillation among those with secondary ventricular fibrillation complicating an acute myocardial infarction was double that among those with primary ventricular fibrillation (P <0.05) (Table 6). Weaver et al. [60] found that a history of congestive heart failure was common in patients with out-of-hospital recurrent ventricular fibrillation/sudden death. They also found that patients with recurrent ventricular fibrillation/sudden death had more triple vessel coronary

16

Table 7. Primary ventricular fibrillation and its recurrence

VF (h)	Patients	RVF
<2	41	6 (15%)*
>2	69	21 (30%)*
Total	110	27 (25%)

* P >0.05
Reproduced with permission [52].

artery disease, lower ejection fractions and more severe abnormalities of left ventricular contraction in comparison with those who had a single episode of ventricular fibrillation and survived during the follow-up period.

4.3. Early and late primary ventricular fibrillation

Of the 141 patients, the initial episode in 110 was primary ventricular fibrillation. The time from the onset of symptoms to the initial episode is shown in Figure 5. Twenty-seven of the 110 patients (25%) had a recurrence (Table 7). The first recurrence occurred at a stage ranging from 38 minutes to 17 days (mean 4 days) after the initial episode of ventricular fibrillation. Of 41 patients with primary ventricular fibrillation within 2 h of an acute myocardial infarction or an acute ischemic episode, 6 (15%) had recurrent ventricular fibrillation and of 69 similar patients with ventricular fibrillation occurring later, 21 (30%) had recurrent ventricular fibrillation. These results did not differ significantly (Table 7). Thus early primary ventricular fibrillation is no more likely to be recurrent than that occurring later (Table 7).

4.4. Non-significant factors

Age, sex, site of infarction, adequacy of initial resuscitation, place of arrest, interval onset of symptoms to initial ventricular fibrillation, onset of symptoms to intensive care, and delay before initial attempted defibrillation were of no significance in the recurrence of ventricular fibrillation. Of the 41 patients with recurrent ventricular fibrillation, 20 patients were receiving antiarrhythmic drugs in what was considered to be therapeutic doses at the time of recurrence of ventricular fibrillation. Nineteen were not receiving antiarrhythmic therapy. The major reasons were the presence of hypotension or heart failure or the delay between the initial episode and its recurrence. In 2 patients the antiarrhythmic therapy was unknown at the time of the recurrence.

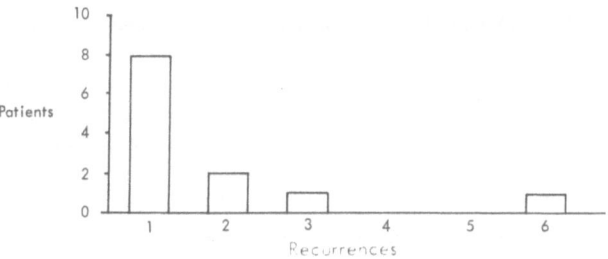

Figure 10. Number of recurrences in the 12 patients with recurrent ventricular fibrillation.

5. RECURRENCE OF VENTRICULAR FIBRILLATION IN EARLY ACUTE MYOCARDIAL INFARCTION

To assess the recurrence of ventricular fibrillation in patients seen at the earliest stage after acute myocardial infarction, a retrospective analysis was carried out of 73 consecutive patients with ventricular fibrillation, managed within one hour of acute myocardial infarction [53]. All patients either had primary ventricular fibrillation at the onset of the acute illness or developed it during hospitalisation. All survived the initial episode of ventricular fibrillation. The period of hospitalisation ranged from 1 to 73 days (mean 23 days). Fifty-six patients (77%) were discharged from hospital. Sixty-four had ventricular fibrillation during the first 12 h from the onset of symptoms: twenty patients were in ventricular fibrillation when first seen (Figure 7).

5.1. Incidence, number and time of recurrence

Twelve of the 73 patients (16%) had recurrent ventricular fibrillation. In 11 of the 12 patients the initial recurrence was primary ventricular fibrillation. Eight of the 12 (67%) had one recurrence while one patient had 6 recurrences (mean 2) (Figure 10). The time interval to recurrent ventricular fibrillation from the initial episode varied from 35 min to 4 days (mean 34 h).

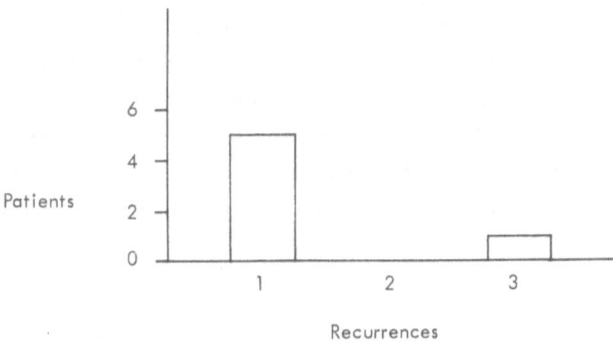

Figure 11. Number of recurrences in the 6 patients with ventricular fibrillation within the first hour.

18

Table 8. Recurrent ventricular fibrillation in patients seen <1 h and >1 h after acute myocardial infarction

(h)	Patients	RVF
<1	73	12 (16%)
>1	58*	13 (22%)

* 58 consecutive patients with primary ventricular fibrillation were managed during 1973–1974. Reproduced with permisson [53].

Ventricular fibrillation occurred within the first hour in 39 of the 73 patients (53%). It recurred in 6 of 39 patients (15%). Five patients had one recurrence and one patient had three recurrences (Figure 11). The time interval from the initial episode to recurrent ventricular fibrillation varied from 1 h to 4 days (mean 43 h).

Thus the incidence of recurrent ventricular fibrillation, the number of recurrences, and the time interval from the initial episode to recurrent ventricular fibrillation were similar whether the initial episode occurred within the first hour of the onset of symptoms or later.

5.2. Early and late primary ventricular fibrillation

In the previous study [52], primary ventricular fibrillation occurring within 2 h of the onset of an acute myocardial infarction or an acute ischemic episode was no more likely to be recurrent than when it occurred later. In this study the incidence of recurrent ventricular fibrillation among patients with primary ventricular fibrillation seen within 1 h of an acute myocardial infarction was similar to comparable patients seen later (Table 8). Thus, the incidence of recurrence was similar whether the initial episode of primary ventricular fibrillation occurred early or late in patients seen within the first hour or later following an acute myocardial infarction.

5.3. Non-significant factors

In the 12 patients with recurrent ventricular fibrillation it was impossible to single out any factor which seemed to put them at extra risk. None of the twelve had bundle branch block or atrioventricular block preceding recurrent ventricular fibrillation. Five of the 12 patients were receiving antiarrhythmic agents in what was considered to be therapeutic doses at the time of the first recurrence. No patient was receiving betablocking agents. Seven patients were not on antiarrhythmic agents. This was mainly due to the time interval between the initial episode of ventricular fibrillation and its recurrence.

REFERENCES

1. Lancisi JM: De Subitaneis Mortibus Libri Duo. Venetiis, 1707.
2. Gordon T, Kannel WB: Premature mortality from coronary heart disease: The Framingham Study. JAMA 215:1617–1625, 1971.
3. Baum RS, Alvarez H, Cobb LA: Survival after resuscitation from out-of-hospital ventricular fibrillation. Circulation 50:1231–1235, 1974.
4. McNamee BT, Robinson TJ, Adgey AAJ, Scott ME, Geddes JS, Pantridge JF: Long-term prognosis following ventricular fibrillation in acute ischaemic heart disease. Br Med J 4:204–206, 1970.
5. Hoffa M, Ludwig C: Einige neue Versuche ueber Herzbewegung. Zeitschrift Fuer Rationelle Medizin 9:107–144, 1850.
6. Abilgard CP: Tentamina electrica in animalibus instituta. Societatis Medicae Havniensis Collectanea 2:157–276, 1775.
7. McWilliam JA: Fibrillar contraction of the heart. J Physiol (Lond) 8:296–310, 1887.
8. McWilliam JA: Cardiac failure and sudden death. Br Med J 1:6–8, 1889.
9. Hoffmann A: Fibrillation of the ventricles at the end of an attack of paroxysmal tachycardia in man. Heart 3:213–217, 1912.
10. Hamilton RL, Robertson H: Electrocardiographic studies of the dying heart in angina pectoris. Can Med Assoc J 29:122–124, 1933.
11. Smith FJ: Ventricular fibrillation as a cause of sudden death in coronary artery thrombosis: report of a case. Am Heart J 17:735–741, 1939.
12. Miller H: Ventricular fibrillation as the mechanism of sudden death in patients with coronary occlusion. N Engl J Med 221:564–569, 1939.
13. Tossach W: Man dead in appearance recovered by distending lungs with air. In: Medical Essays and Observations, Volume 5, Part 2, p. 108. Cadell T, Balfour J, eds. London and Edinburgh, 1771.
14. Kouwenhoven WB, Jude JR, Knickerbocker GG: Closed-chest cardiac massage. JAMA 173: 1064–1067, 1960.
15. Cole SL, Corday E: Four-minute limit for cardiac resuscitation. JAMA 161:1454–1458, 1956.
16. Prevost JL, Battelli F: La mort par les courants electriques: Courants alternatifs a haute tension. (Death by electric currents alternating at high tension). Journal de Physiologie et de Pathologie Generale 1:427–441, 1899.
17. Hooker DR, Kouwenhoven WB, Langworthy OR: The effect of alternating electrical currents on the heart. Am J Physiol 103:444–454, 1933.
18. Beck CS, Pritchard WH, Feil HS: Ventricular fibrillation of long duration abolished by electric shock. JAMA 135:985–986, 1947.
19. Weinberger LM, Gibbon MH, Gibbon JH Jr: Temporary arrest of the circulation to the central nervous system: 1: Physiologic effects. Arch Neurol Psychiatr 43:615–634, 1940.
20. Reagan LB, Young KR, Nicholson JW: Ventricular defibrillation in a patient with probable acute coronary occlusion. Surgery 39:482–486, 1956.
21. Beck CS, Weckesser EC, Barry FM: Fatal heart attack and successful defibrillation: new concepts in coronary artery disease. JAMA 161:434–436, 1956.
22. Straight WM, Litwak R, Turner JC Jr: Sudden death in acute myocardial infarction: report of a case, with observations on the cause, prevention and management. Ann Int Med 54:566–582, 1961.
23. Brass PR, Kendell RE: Successful cardiac massage after myocardial infarction in a casualty department. Br Med J 1:26–29, 1961.
24. Burns A: Observations on disease of the coronary arteries and on syncope anginosa. In: Observations on Some of the Most Frequent and Important Diseases of the Heart, p. 147. Edinburgh: Muirhead J, 1809.
25. Ferris LP, King BG, Spence PW, Williams HB: Effect of electric shock on heart. Electric Eng 55:498–515, 1936.

26. Gurvich NL, Yuniev GS: Restoration of regular rhythm in mammalian fibrillating heart. Am Rev Sov Med 3:236–239, 1946.
27. Gurvich NL, Yuniev GA: Restoration of heart rhythm during fibrillation by condenser discharge. Am Rev Sov Med 4:252–256, 1947.
28. Zoll PM, Linenthal AJ, Gibson W, Paul MH, Norman LR: Termination of ventricular fibrillation in man by externally applied electric countershock. N Engl J Med 254:727–732, 1956.
29. Lown B, Neuman J, Amarasingham R, Berkovits BV: Comparison of alternating current with direct current electroshock across the closed chest. Am J Cardiol 10:223–233, 1962.
30. Pantridge JF, Geddes JS: Cardiac arrest after myocardial infarction. Lancet i:807–808, 1966.
31. Pantridge JF, Geddes JS: A mobile intensive-care unit in the management of myocardial infarction. Lancet ii:271–273, 1967.
32. Zipes DP, Fischer J, King RM, Nicoll ADB, Jolly WW: Termination of ventricular fibrillation in dogs by depolarising a critical amount of myocardium. Am J Cardiol 36:37–44, 1975.
33. Tacker WA Jr, Galioto FM Jr, Giuliani E, Geddes LA, McNamara DG: Energy dosage for human trans-chest electrical ventricular defibrillation. N Engl J Med 290:214–215, 1974.
34. Tacker WA Jr, Geddes LA: Ventricular defibrillation. Br J Clin Equipm 2:13–18, 1977.
35. Campbell NPS, Webb SW, Adgey AAJ, Pantridge JF: Transthoracic ventricular defibrillation in adults. Br Med J 2:1379–1381, 1977.
36. Gascho JA, Crampton RS, Cherwek ML, Sipes JN, Hunter FP, O'Brien WM: Determinants of ventricular defibrillation in adults. Circulation 60:231–240, 1979.
37. Kerber RE, Sarnat W: Factors influencing the success of ventricular defibrillation in man. Circulation 60:226–230, 1979.
38. Geddes LA: Damped sinusoidal waveforms for ventricular defibrillation. Presented at the Cardiac Defibrillation Conference, p. 55. West Lafayette, Ind: Purdue University, 1975.
39. Curry JJ, Quintana FJ: Myocardial infarction with ventricular fibrillation during pregnancy treated by direct current defibrillation with fetal survival. Chest 58:82–84, 1970.
40. Lappin HA: Ventricular defibrillators in heavy patients. N Engl J Med 291:153, 1974.
41. Tacker WA Jr, Morris GC, Winters WL: Transchest ventricular defibrillation of a subject weighing 102.5 kg (225.9 lbs). South Med J 68:786–788, 1975.
42. DeSilva RA, Lown B: Energy requirement for defibrillation of a markedly overweight patient. Circulation 57:827–830, 1978.
43. Gascho JA, Crampton RS, Sipes JN, Cherwek ML, Hunter FP, O'Brien WM: Energy levels and patient weight in ventricular defibrillation. JAMA 242:1380–1384, 1979.
44. Collins RE, Giuliani ER, Tacker WA Jr, Geddes LA: Transthoracic ventricular defibrillation: success and body weight. Med Instrum 12:53, 1978 (abstract).
45. Anderson GJ, Suelzer J: The efficacy of trapezoidal wave forms for ventricular defibrillation. Chest 70:298–300, 1976.
46. Tacker WA Jr, Guinn GA, Geddes LA, Bourland JD, Korompai FL, Rubio PA: The electrical dose for direct ventricular defibrillation in man. J Thorac Cardiovasc Surg 75:224–226, 1978.
47. Rubio PA, Farrell EM: Low-energy direct defibrillation of the human heart. Ann Thorac Surg 27:32–33, 1979.
48. Geddes LA, Tacker WA Jr, Rosborough JP, Moore AG, Cabler PS: Electrical dose for ventricular defibrillation of large and small animals using precordial electrodes. J Clin Invest 53:310–319, 1974.
49. Pantridge JF, Webb SW, Adgey AAJ: Arrhythmias in the first hours of acute myocardial infarction. Prog Cardiovasc Dis 23:265–278, 1981.
50. Patton JN, Allen JD, Pantridge JF: Myocardial damage from transthoracic DC shocks. Presented at Third Purdue Conference on Cardiac Defibrillation and Cardiopulmonary Resuscitation. Purdue University, West Lafayette, Ind., 1979.
51. Weaver WD, Thurman C, Copass MK, Hallstrom AP, Cobb LA: Ventricular defibrillation. A prospective comparative trial of 175 joule and 320 joule energies. p. 108. Proceedings: Association for the Advancement of Medical Instrumentation, Washington DC, 1981 (abstract).

52. Logan KR, McIlwaine WJ, Adgey AAJ, Pantridge JF: Recurrence of ventricular fibrillation in acute ischemic heart disease. Circulation, 64:1163–1167, 1981.
53. Logan KR, McIlwaine WJ, Adgey AAJ, Pantridge JF: Ventricular fibrillation and its recurrence in early acute myocardial infarction. Lancet 1:242–244, 1981.
54. Lie KI, Wellens HJ, Durrer D: Characteristics and predictability of primary ventricular fibrillation. Eur J Cardiol 1:379–384, 1974.
55. Lie KI, Durrer D: Ventricular fibrillation and acute myocardial infarction. Compr Ther 3:16–19, 1977.
56. El-Sherif N, Myerburg RJ, Scherlag BJ, Befeler B, Aranda JM, Castellanos A, Lazzara R: Electro-cardiographic antecedents of primary ventricular fibrillation. Value of the R-on-T phenomenon in myocardial infarction. Br Heart J 38:415–422, 1976.
57. Cobb LA, Baum RS, Alvarez H III, Schaffer WA: Resuscitation from out-of-hospital ventricular fibrillation: 4 years follow-up. Circulation 51 & 52 (suppl III):III-223–III-228, 1975.
58. Schaffer WA, Cobb LA: Recurrent ventricular fibrillation and modes of death in survivors of out-of-hospital ventricular fibrillation. N Engl J Med 293:259–262, 1975.
59. Haynes RE, Hallstrom AP, Cobb LA: Repolarization abnormalities in survivors of out-of-hospital ventricular fibrillation. Circulation 57:654–658, 1978.
60. Weaver WD, Lorch GS, Alvarez HA, Cobb LA: Angiographic findings and prognostic indicators in patients resuscitated from sudden cardiac death. Circulation 54:895–900, 1976

2. A NEW LOOK AT CARDIOPULMONARY RESUSCITATION

STEVEN UNG, JAMES T. NIEMANN and J. MICHAEL CRILEY

1. INTRODUCTION

Although the development of Coronary Care Units has resulted in a 30% reduction in mortality among hospitalized patients with acute myocardial infarction [1], approximately two-thirds of patients who die from coronary heart disease do not reach a hospital [1–3]. Sudden death in these patients with atherosclerotic heart disease has been attributed to ventricular arrhythmias or ventricular fibrillation. In this setting, the time between the onset of arrest and initiation of resuscitative measures is critical if mortality and morbidity is to be minimized.

Bystander-initiated cardiopulmonary resuscitation (CPR) has become the crucial link in maintaining vital organ perfusion while help is being summoned [4]. Yet despite the rapidity with which CPR may be initiated by the laity, the survival statistics for out-of-hospital arrest have been less than optimal. An objective re-evaluation of basic CPR and its improvement have been overshadowed by the major emphasis directed towards prevention of sudden death: identification of high risk patients, definition of potential causes, and new advances in antiarrhythmic therapy. However, as we have come to recognize that improving blood flow during CPR in these victims might be a means of improving survival while awaiting electrical defibrillation and advanced life support, there has been a renewed interest in the mechanical aspects and mechanism of blood flow during closed-chest CPR.

This chapter will review the mechanism(s) of blood flow during CPR and the research being conducted towards improving the technique as it is practised in the field. But to understand the present status and future of CPR, one must first review its historical development.

2. HISTORICAL PERSPECTIVE

For centuries man has been interested in cardiac resuscitation [5, 6]. Records in the early 17th century document pioneering animal research by physiologists and physicians in this field. Because the heart was then considered the center of the circulation and the 'seat of the spirit of life', those early attempts at restoration of the circulation focused on restoring the 'pumping action' of the heart. In 1895, the technique of open chest cardiac massage was first described by a physiologist,

Adgey, AAJ (ed): Acute phase of ischemic heart disease and myocardial infarction.
© *1982, Martinus Nijhoff, The Hague, Boston, London. ISBN-13: 978-94-009-7581-1*

Mortiz Schiff, in a dog who had succumbed during chloroform anesthesia. Several years later and with subsequent modification, this technique was applied to man, and the 'subcostal or subdiaphragmatic' approach to opening the thorax and the direct massaging/compressing of the arrested heart became an accepted and standard method of cardiac resuscitation during the early decades of this century [6]. The technique, however, had an obvious limitation in that it could be applied only by those with a medical background and training.

Although 'indirect' cardiac massage by thoracic compression was first performed in man and reported in the late 1780's by John Hovard [5], the development of 'indirect' cardiac massage remained in the background of open-chest cardiac massage until its rediscovery in 1960 by Dr. Kouwenhoven and associates at The Johns Hopkins University [7, 8]. Dr. Kouwenhoven, an Emeritus Professor of Engineering at the University, was then working on a method for external defibrillation of electrical linemen and other workers who were dying of accidental electrocution [8]. One of the safety devices of the electrodes for the portable DC defibrillator his group was using was the requirement for at least 12 pounds of pressure by the electrodes on the chest before activation of the switch could occur. They astutely noted that a rise in arterial blood pressure could be generated from that forceful application of the electrodes, even before countershock was delivered. Their experiments subsequent to that observation led to their now famous publication and prescription for 'closed-chest cardiac massage' [7]. Combined with the technique of artificial respiration, closed-chest cardiac massage was adopted over open-chest cardiac massage as the standard for cardiopulmonary resuscitation, since 'anyone, anywhere could initiate CPR with the help of two hands'.

The mechanism of how CPR operated was felt to be quite simple. Because of its anatomic location, Kouwenhoven and coworkers believed that the heart was compressed between sternum and spine during each chest compression, producing a 'cardiac pump' that generated forward blood flow [7]. Implicit in this explanation were the requirements for functioning, competent atrioventricular valves and an arteriovenous gradient during compression to allow for unidirectional blood flow. Although the technique gained clinical acceptance, there was a paucity of scientific data to support this mechanism. In fact, as investigators studied the mechanism of blood flow and attempted to quantitate blood flow during chest compression compared to other resuscitative measures (e.g. open-chest cardiac massage), several conflicting observations were made that suggested the mechanism of blood flow not to be as simple as previously thought.

In 1962, Weale and Rothwell-Jackson [9] demonstrated equalization of venous and arterial pressures during chest compression in fibrillating dogs. They interpreted these data as indicating atrioventricular valve incompetence and concluded that chest compression resulted in a global increase in intrathoracic pressures with resultant bidirectional transmission of pressure pulses in the arterial and venous beds. Figure 1 demonstrates simultaneous recordings of aortic, and right and left atrial pressures in a dog during CPR in our laboratory, and reveals equal 'systolic'

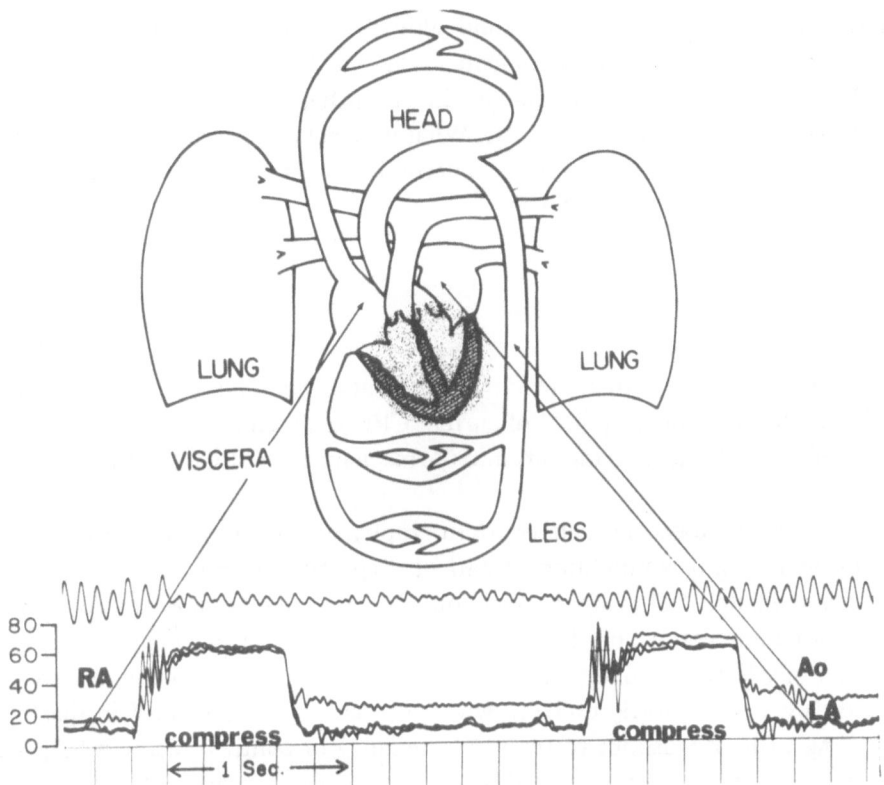

Figure 1. Systemic arterial and atrial pressures generated by external chest compression.

Simultaneous equisensitive pressure recordings from a dog in ventricular fibrillation undergoing chest compressions at a slow rate, reveal equal pressures during compression in the aorta (Ao) and both atria. If selective ventricular compression (shaded area) were responsible for blood flow in CPR, it would be anticipated that the atrial pressures are lower than arterial pressure. Because of the equal 'systolic' pressures in the aorta and right atrium (RA), there is no apparent systolic arteriovenous gradient to produce flow through the systemic vascular bed. There is a small diastolic arterioatrial gradient due to arterial tonus.

pressures from all three locations. Similar observations were made by others who were equally perplexed about the mechanism of forward blood flow in the absence of a demonstrable atrioventricular gradient [10, 11]. They also suggested that during chest compression, the high venous pressures might be transmitted to the cerebral and pulmonary circulations. These high venous pressures could theoretically reverse the normal arteriovenous capillary gradient, resulting in impaired blood flow in the respective vascular beds.

Clinical observations by others [12] cast further doubt on the cardiac pump mechanism, as they noted that closed-chest cardiac massage was successful in emphysematous patients with increased anteroposterior diameters which makes direct cardiac compression unlikely. Furthermore, they failed to obtain adequate arterial pressures in patients with flail chests during chest compression, a situation in which a flail sternum should allow easy compression of the heart.

By the late 1960's enough experimental data and clinical observations had been made to cast suspicion and doubt on direct cardiac compression as being the mechanism of blood flow during CPR. What was lacking was an observation that could organize these findings into an alternative theory. The observations from 'Cough CPR' provided that catalyst.

3. COUGH CPR

Cough CPR is an interesting phenomenon the understanding and recognition of which paralleled the development of current CPR research and consequently provided many useful clues and insights into the mechanism of blood flow during CPR [13].

During the early days of coronary arteriography, coughing was used as a method to improve the clinical condition of patients experiencing bradycardia or hypotension immediately following the injection of contrast material. It was not understood how cough worked, but Dr. Mason Sones, a pioneer in cineangiography and developer of selective coronary arteriography, had postulated that cough caused a marked elevation of aortic pressure when the ventricle was relaxed in diastole, facilitating prompt washout of the small quantity of contrast medium [14]. Although this notion is still propagated [15], subsequent experience with cough in the cardiac catheterization laboratory has shown that this explanation is too simplistic.

In 1976 our laboratory published a report detailing hemodynamic observations of vigorous coughing in patients experiencing cardiac arrest while undergoing cardiac catheterization [16]. The salient feature of these patients was that coughing could maintain adequate arterial pressure and consciousness until definitive therapy, in most cases electrical defibrillation, was rendered. It appeared that in selected patients, coughing during ventricular fibrillation or asystole could produce blood flow and serve as an alternative to conventional CPR. This method was termed 'Cough CPR.'

The hemodynamic data from a representative case are presented in Figure 2. This was a patient in whom ventricular fibrillation developed as he was undergoing coronary arteriography. Following the onset of fibrillation, the patient was instructed to cough vigorously. During the 39 s of coughing it took to get the defibrillation paddles in place and apply countershock, an arterial pressure of 130–140 mm Hg was generated with each cough and the patient maintained consciousness. Clearly cough was producing substantial aortic pressures and maintaining consciousness.

Nonetheless, questions were raised whether the cough-induced aortic pressures represented actual cardiac output if consciousness could be maintained without coughing and, most importantly, what the mechanism was by which cough-CPR

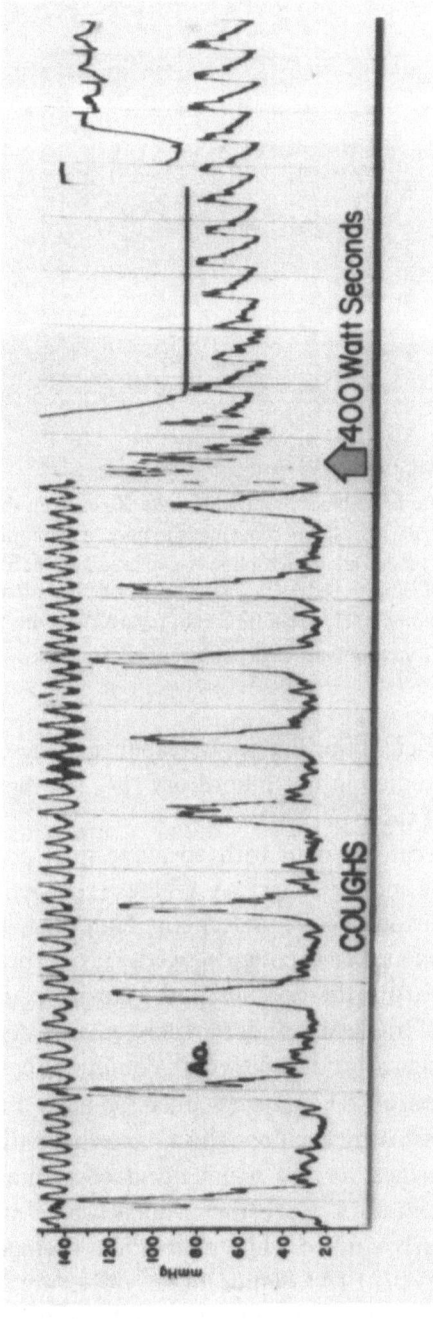

Figure 2. Cough CPR during ventricular fibrillation in man.

A 43-year-old man postoperative from coronary bypass surgery developed ventricular fibrillation during coronary arteriography and was instructed to cough vigorously while preparations were made to perform countershock. Central aortic pressure recording demonstrated average peak systolic pressure of 140 mmHg with coughs, and he remained conscious throughout the 39-s episode of ventricular fibrillation. He reverted to sinus rhythm after a single 400 Ws countershock. (Time lines = 1 s.)

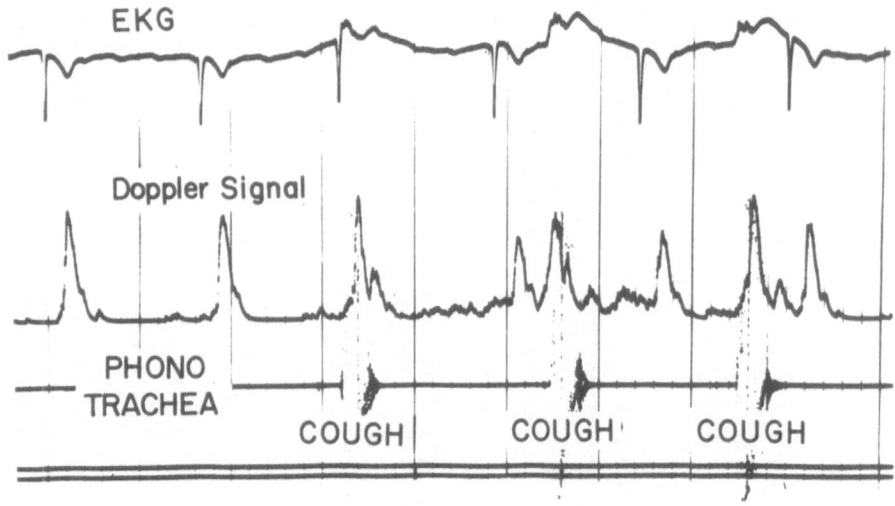

Figure 3. Cough CPR during complete heart block.

A 49-year-old man developed complete heart block, ventricular rate 38, early in the course of an inferior wall myocardial infarction. As preparations were being made to insert a temporary transvenous pacemaker, he was asked to cough several times while a microphone was placed over the trachea to record coughs and an external Doppler flow-velocity probe was placed over the brachial artery. Each cough produced a brachial flow-velocity signal comparable to control beats, regardless of the 'prematurity' of the cough relative to the beats resulting from spontaneous depolarization. (Time lines = 1 s.)

produced blood flow during ventricular fibrillation. In response to these challenges, another group of patients was studied in our laboratory [17, 18]. Again, the following cases are representative of those patients.

The first case involved a 49-year-old man with an acute inferior myocardial infarction complicated by syncope and high degree A-V block (ventricular response 38/min despite isoproterenol infusion). While undergoing temporary transvenous pacemaker insertion, the patient was asked to cough between his own beats. Figure 3 depicts the EKG, analog signal from the doppler flow velocity probe over the brachial artery, and phonogram of tracheal sounds to record coughs. As can be seen in the tracings, the flow velocity signal produced by each cough was comparable in amplitude to the signal produced by the patient's intrinsic beat. Furthermore, neither was the blood flow produced by each cough influenced by the preceding spontaneous beat, nor did it influence the flow which occurred with a subsequent spontaneous beat. Another patient with a prosthetic aortic valve and a failing permanent pacemaker was similarly studied while undergoing exchange of pacemaker generators. Figure 4 shows the EKG, femoral artery pressure and doppler flow velocity signal from a transducer placed over the brachial artery. Simultaneous cinefluoroscopy permitted visualization of the opening movement of the prosthetic valve poppet. Each cough produced a pressure and flow signal (A) as well as aortic valve opening. Each cough was followed by a ventricular depolarization which

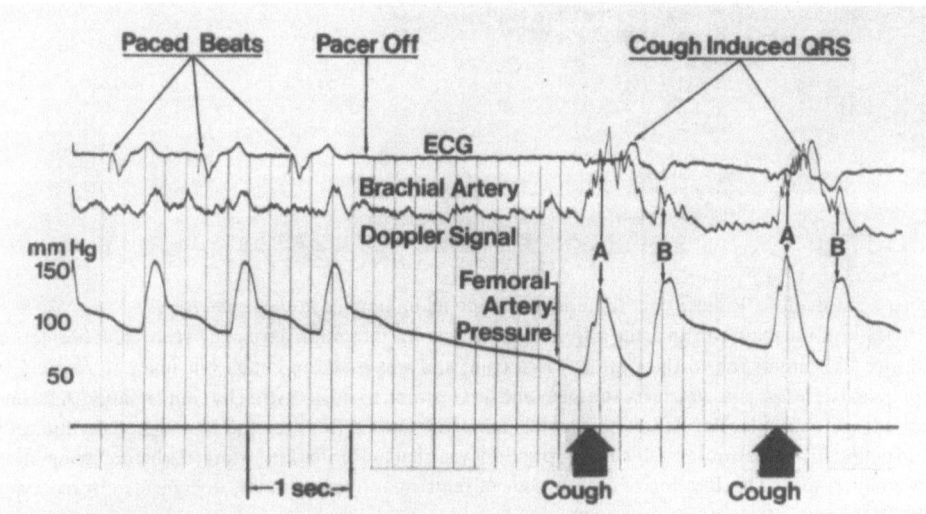

Figure 4. Cough CPR during pacemaker-dependent heart block.

A 36-year-old male postoperative from aortic valve replacement and permanent pacemaker was noted to be completely pacemaker-dependent when the electrode leads were removed from the pacemaker generator at the time of exchange of the unit. During monitoring of the femoral artery pressure and brachial artery Doppler signal, he was asked to cough as the pacemaker generator was exchanged. The first cough produced an arterial pulse pressure and flow signal larger than the control beats. Following the cough-induced pressure and flow, a QRS complex occurred and resulted in another pressure and flow pulse despite its 'premature' position. Because each cough-induced pulse was reproducibly followed by a QRS complex and cardiac contraction, it was assumed that ventricular depolarization was mechanically stimulated by the cough. (Time lines = 1 s.)

produced an additional pressure and flow signal (B) and opening of the aortic valve.

The third case supported the contention that cerebral blood flow occurred during coughing. The patient was a 53-year-old male with an acute inferior myocardial infarction. Within two hours of hospitalization primary ventricular fibrillation occurred (Figure 5). Conventional CPR was instituted and the patient regained consciousness following cardioversion. Shortly thereafter, he suffered a second episode of ventricular fibrillation but was able to respond to instructions to cough. With vigorous coughing he was able to maintain consciousness for 92 s before countershock could be delivered. Because he had acted as his own control, it appeared that coughing could maintain the cerebral circulation without any other form of circulatory assistance.

In the experimental laboratory these results were confirmed by a 'coughing dog' model developed by Dr. Rosborough and associates [18]. Preparation of this model involved anesthetizing a dog with intravenous ketamine, intubating the animal, and placing electrodes on both of the cervical vagosympathetic nerve trunks. Following induction of ventricular fibrillation, electrical stimulation of the cervical nerve trunks induced paroxysms of coughing. To create a cough of comparable duration

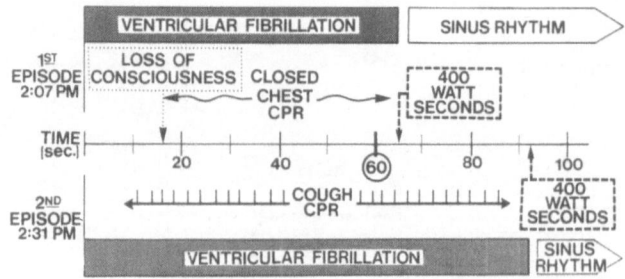

Figure 5. Cough CPR during ventricular fibrillation maintaining consciousness for 92 s.

A 53-year-old man with an acute inferior wall myocardial infarction developed ventricular fibrillation shortly after admission to the Cardiac Care Unit, and was asked to cough but failed to respond to commands. He lost consciousness 16 s later, and was restored to sinus rhythm by countershock. A second episode of ventricular fibrillation occurred 24 min later, and on this occasion he coughed rhythmically and maintained consciousness during an episode of ventricular fibrillation lasting 92 s before termination by countershock. The duration of each episode of ventricular fibrillation was documented by replaying the electrocardiogram stored on magnetic tape.

to that of a human cough, the endotracheal tube was briefly occluded to simulate glottal action. Figure 6 illustrates hemodynamic measurements obtained during ventricular fibrillation in a coughing dog preparation.

Left ventricular and aortic pressures rose simultaneously during cough with the average peak systolic pressure generated by the cough being 75 mm Hg. Cineangio-

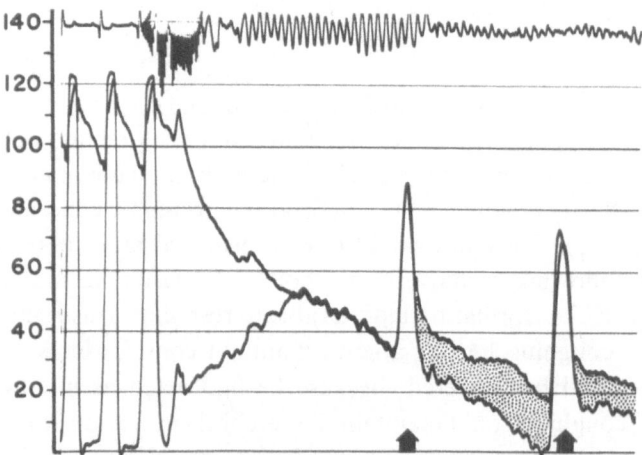

Figure 6. Cough CPR during ventricular fibrillation in a dog.

Using Rosborough's technique of emulating coughing in a dog instrumented with micromanometer catheters in the left ventricle and aorta, ventricular fibrillation is induced and the aortic and left ventricular pressures equilibrate and then decline. With each cough (arrow) a pressure pulse averaging 75 mm Hg is produced in the left ventricle, and there is a diastolic pressure gradient (shaded area) due to arterial tonus. Cineangiograms of this dog (see Figure 7) revealed aortic valve opening with each cough. (Time lines = 1 s.)

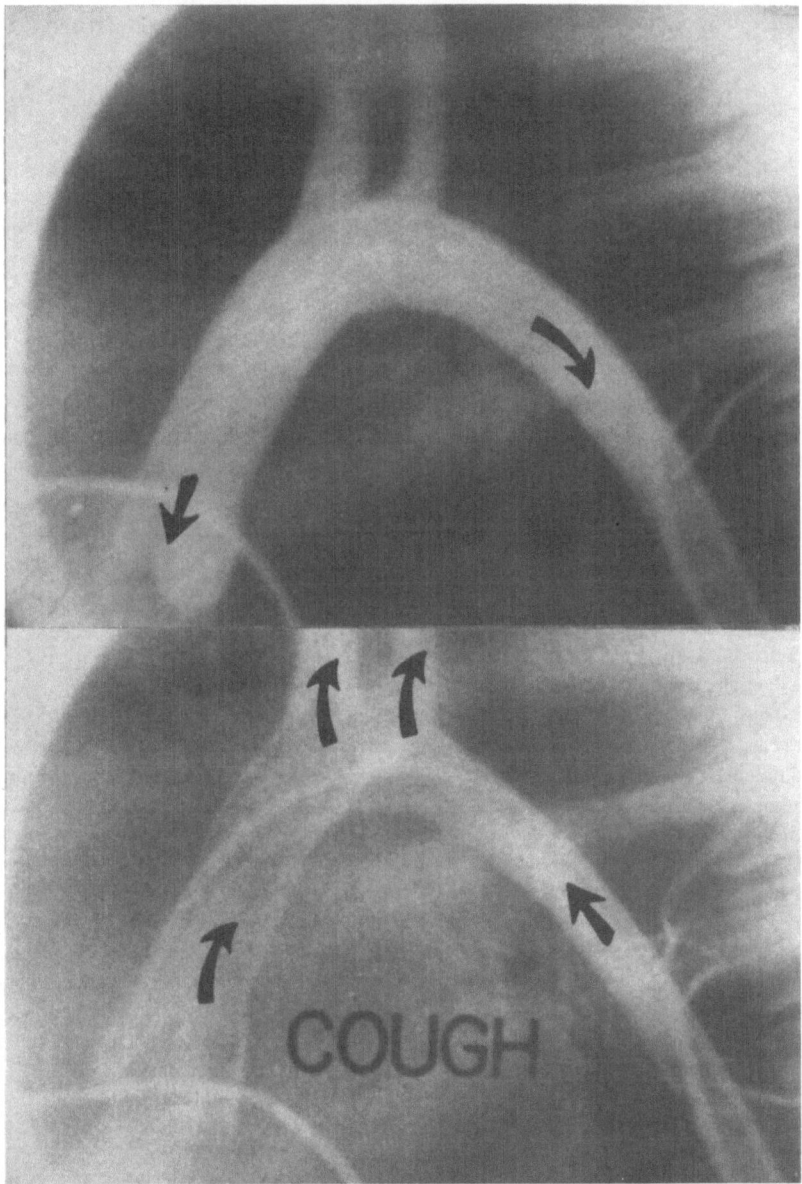

Figure 7. Aortography during cough CPR in a dog with ventricular fibrillation.

An injection of contrast medium has been made in the descending aorta during ventricular fibrillation. Early 'diastole' following the first cough (upper panel) demonstrates a closed aortic valve, and flow was seen on motion analysis to move towards the aortic valve in the ascending aorta and towards the abdominal aorta from the descending aorta (arrows).

In the lower panel, taken during 'cough systole', the aortic valve has opened and flow of contrast medium occurs towards the brachiocephalic vessels from both the ascending and descending aorta (arrows). Opacification of the left ventricle can be seen in the lower left corner, which resulted from aortic regurgitation during the previous 'cough diastole'.

32

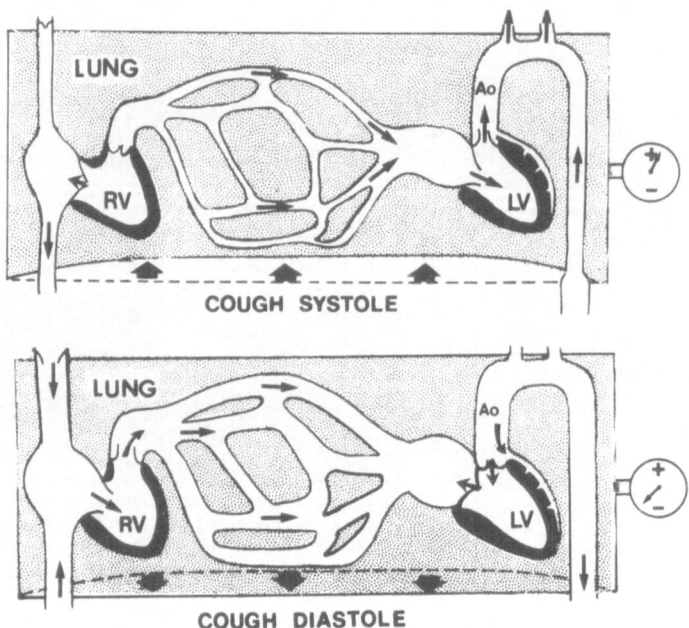

Figure 8. The mechanism of flow in cough CPR.

These diagrams are based on hemodynamic and cineangiographic studies of cough CPR in the dog. The thorax is represented as a rectangular compartment containing the lungs (shaded areas), the right and left heart, and the intervening pulmonary vascular bed. Positive and negative pressure events are depicted by a dial manometer on the right. During 'cough systole', the pressure in the thorax is increased abruptly, closing the venous valves at the thoracic inlet and squeezing the aorta to initiate flow through the brachiocephalic vessels. Blood is then milked from the pulmonary vessels through both of the left heart chambers to exit the thorax preferentially through the brachiocephalic arteries. The high abdominal pressure generated by the contraction of abdominal wall muscles during cough inhibits subdiaphragmatic flow, and the low jugular venous pressure (see Figure 12) enhances brachiocephalic flow. In the right heart, the pulmonic valve closes competently, but the tricuspid valve is incompetent. Reflux occurs to a greater degree into the inferior vena cava because closure of the superior thoracic inlet venous valves inhibits cephalad venous flow.

During 'cough diastole', venous inflow through the right heart occurs augmented by the negative pressure of pre-cough inspiration. In the left heart, the mitral and aortic valves are incompetent. Some coronary flow is seen, and descending aortic blood flows into the abdominal aorta (see Figure 7).

grams with aortic root contrast injections during the cough–fibrillation period demonstrated several interesting observations. During ventricular fibrillation the aortic and mitral valves were incompletely closed and valvar regurgitation was present in all cases. Anterograde blood flow occurred with each cough, with preferential flow to the brachiocephalic circulation (Figure 7). This preferential flow was felt to be due to the inhibition of flow to the abdominal aorta by the increased intra-abdominal pressure during active coughing (see below for mechanism of cough). Both the mitral and aortic valves are opened during the high pressure phase of each cough with an average anterograde transaortic valve flow duration of over 200 ms, as determined angiographically. There is no visible evidence of cardiac compression, but instead the pulmonary veins appear to be compressed with each cough, 'milking' blood through the left heart. In these experiments the left heart was therefore a passive conduit for blood expressed from the pulmonary vascular bed to the systemic arteries.

These observations in man and animals confirmed that in the absence of chest compression, cough could: 1) generate hemodynamically significant forward blood flow; 2) produce an arterial pressure pulse; 3) open the aortic valve; and 4) maintain consciousness during circulatory arrest. The mechanism by which this all occurred was postulated to involve the phasic changes in developed intrathoracic pressures during cough [18].

Cough CPR can de divided into two phases or cycles based on changes in intrathoracic pressure and dynamic blood flow. The first phase has been called 'cough systole' (Figure 8). Contraction of the intercostal and abdominal muscles at the onset of cough generates a pressure of about 100-180 mm Hg against a closed glottis for a period of approximately 0.2 s (19). Compression of intrathoracic contents occurs, after which the glottis is opened and air forcefully expelled, relieving the elevated intrathoracic pressure. The increased intrathoracic pressure is believed to force blood from the intrathoracic vascular structures into the lower-pressure extrathoracic vessels. Since the left atrial, the left ventricular, and the aortic pressures rise to the same level during cough, the ventricle cannot be selectively compressed. Thus, during cough the left ventricle acts as a passive conduit with one-way valves and the thorax becomes the 'pump' with a potential reservoir equal to the pulmonary blood volume, 200–300 ml/M^2 [20]. From this reservoir, an adequate 'stroke volume' can be obtained.

The second phase of cough and cough CPR begins when the intrathoracic pressure falls and is therefore called 'cough diastole' (see Figure 8). As the intrathoracic pressure declines, the aortic valve closes, thereby maintaining a diastolic pressure gradient as required for coronary perfusion. A simultaneous fall in intra-abdominal pressure caused by muscle relaxation facilitates subdiaphragmatic blood flow. For a subsequent forceful cough to occur, a deep precough inspiration is taken and this inspiration generates a negative intrathoracic pressure of − 10 to − 20 mm Hg [20]. There is angiographic evidence [21] that this deep precough inspiration accelerates venous return through the right heart to the pulmonary vasculature and thus 'primes the pump' for the ensuing cough.

Cough CPR has obvious inherent limitations with respect to its practical applicability. The individual must have prior instruction, be aware or be warned of his impending ventricular fibrillation, and be awake to implement the coughing. With such prerequisites, it is probably most suitable for the controlled environment of the cardiac catheterization laboratory or the coronary care unit. However, aside from its practical utility, the greatest significance of cough CPR is to provide a window to a possible mechanism of blood flow during conventional CPR by demonstrating a means by which blood flowed without direct cardiac compression.

4. MECHANISM OF BLOOD FLOW IN CPR

Although the mechanism of blood flow during CPR has been attributed to cardiac compression, simulating open-chest cardiac massage, there is mounting experimental and clinical evidence, in addition to the observations of cough CPR, that seriously questions the traditional 'cardiac pump' mechanism as the sole impetus for blood flow during CPR.

If cardiac compression were the driving force for blood flow during CPR, it would be expected that the ventricles are compressed more or less selectively in order for the 'cardiac pump' to function efficiently. This forward flow would require a positive arteriovenous pressure gradient, that is, a higher pressure in the aorta and pulmonary arteries than in the right and left atria, respectively.

Since numerous observations in man and animals have failed to demonstrate this expected gradient between the aorta and right atrium, and have instead demonstrated equal pressure rises in the aorta and both atria during chest compression, the prerequisites for an efficient 'cardiac pump' seem not to be present during CPR. The marked discrepancy between the expected and observed pressure events led several investigative groups, including our laboratory, to attempt to document the mechanism(s) by which blood flows during CPR.

4.1. Left heart studies during CPR

Cineangiography of experimental animals during ventricular fibrillation revealed incomplete closure of the cardiac valves with appearance of contrast media in the left ventricle and left atrium when injected manually in the aortic root. During sternal depression (CPR 'systole'), forward flow is initiated in the aortic root before the aortic valve is seen to open, following which anterograde flow is seen to traverse the two left heart valves as both the mitral and aortic valves open widely. Two-dimensional echocardiographic studies by Werner and coworkers in patients during cardiac arrest have also demonstrated that the partially closed mitral valve opens more widely during chest compression at the time when the aortic valve opens [22].

When radio-opaque oil droplets are used as 'tracer bullets' to follow the timing and direction of blood flow during CPR, manual injections into the pulmonary veins demonstrate forward flow of the opaque markers through both left heart chambers during a single compression, and preferential flow to the brachiocephalic arteries. These cineangiographic findings are similar to the observations made during 'cough CPR' but the magnitude of flow appeared to be significantly less during chest compression.

To quantitate the differences in magnitude of flow, cannulating electromagnetic flow probes were placed in the carotid arteries to compare 'cough CPR' and chest compression CPR. Cough produced approximately 40% of control (sinus rhythm) carotid blood flow, while chest compression yielded approximately 10% of control flow. Utilizing simultaneous chest compression and lung inflation, as proposed by

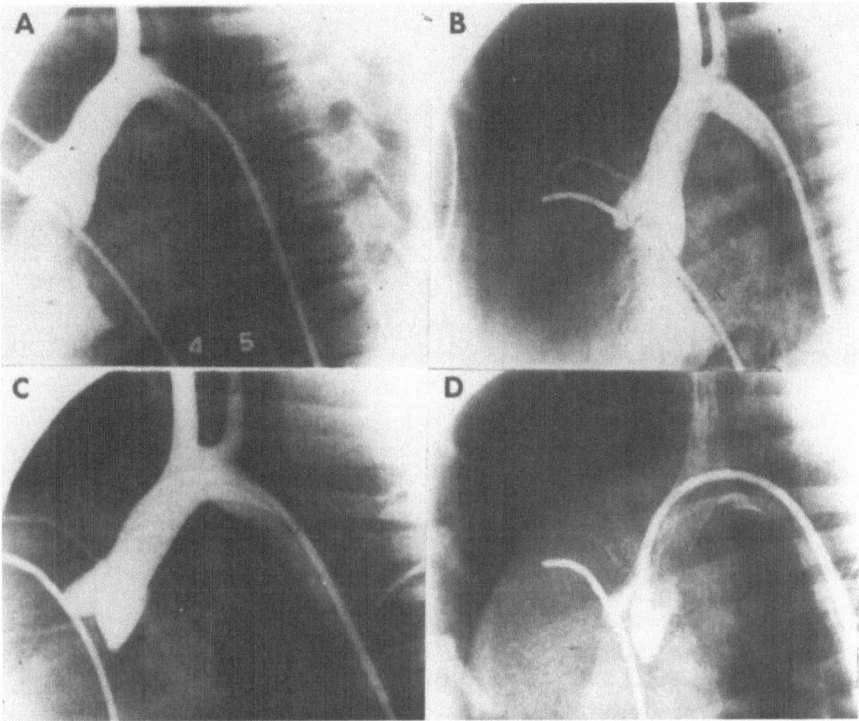

Figure 9. Aortography during CPR in the dog; the effect of simultaneous compression and inflation.

Panels A and B demonstrate relaxation and 2.5 inch standard CPR compression following an aortic root injection of contrast medium in a dog in ventricular fibrillation. Aortic regurgitation is seen with opacification of the left ventricle in both panels. During compression (B), the heart and aorta have been displaced dorsally, there is greater opacification of the brachiocephalic arteries at the apex of the aortic arch, and very little flow is seen towards the descending aorta.

Panels C and D demonstrate relaxation and 2.5 inch compression after lung inflation. There is less aortic regurgitation, and better clearance of contrast medium indicating greater flow. The augmentation of forward flow by simultaneous inflation and compression was confirmed by flow probe recordings from the carotid arteries.

Weisfeldt's group [12], carotid blood flow could be doubled to approximately 20% of control flow. Other modifications such as abdominal binding and negative pulmonary pressure between compressions can further increase the carotid blood flow.

Cineangiographic studies during simultaneous chest compression and lung inflation demonstrated dramatic increases in the magnitude of forward flow of the contrast media as well as less aortic valvar regurgitation between compressions (Figure 9). In none of the cineangiographic studies was significant ventricular compression demonstrated. When the force and depth of compression of the chest was purposely increased in order to achieve ventricular compression, the heart was seen to roll off the spine towards the left hemithorax; also, the magnitude of forward

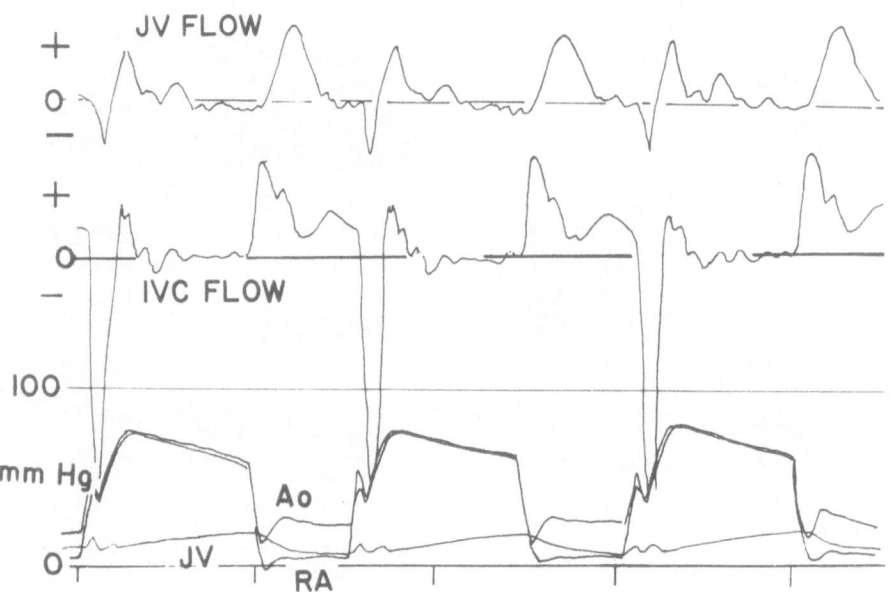

Figure 10. Venous flow during CPR in the dog with ventricular fibrillation.

Cannulating flow probes have been inserted into the abdominal inferior vena cava (IVC) and jugular vein (JV), and equisensitive micromanometer catheters have been placed in the aorta (Ao), Jugular vein (JV), and right atrium (RA), and recordings made during chest compressions at 45 compressions/min. Flow towards the heart is indicated with a plus sign, while reflux is below baseline, or negative. During compression, indicated by abrupt pressure increases to 75 mm Hg in the aortic and right atrial pressure tracings, there is a lesser rise in the jugular venous pressure because of the interposition of a venous valve (see Figure 11). Flow signals reveal marked early systolic reflux in the inferior vena cava and a lesser quantity and duration of reflux in the jugular vein. Flow towards the heart occurs during release of compression. The small amount of positive flow seen during compression is probably an artifact caused by movement of the vascular structures during chest compression, since it is not seen by cineangiography. (Time lines = 1 s.)

flow decreased and the degree of aortic regurgitation increased. It was assumed that the distortion of the heart and valves actually obstructed the left heart conduit.

4.2. The right heart in CPR

Right heart cineangiographic studies during CPR in fibrillating dogs have revealed that most of the observed pulmonary flow is out of phase with aortic flow, occurring during the relaxation phase between compressions [23]. Sternal depression initially causes a small forward surge of blood through the pulmonic valve, but there is a concomitant major reflux from the right ventricle and right atrium into the great veins, particularly the inferior vena cava. Shortly after the completion of sternal depression, the pulmonic valve closes and remains closed throughout the duration of the compression phase.

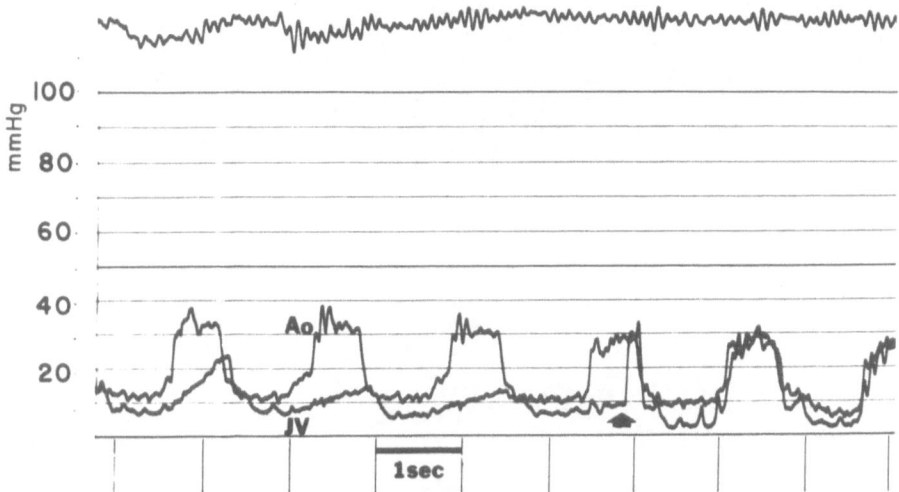

Figure 11A. Hemodynamic demonstration of thoracic inlet venous valve.

Micromanometer catheters have been placed in the aorta (Ao) and jugular vein (JV) in a dog with ventricular fibrillation undergoing CPR. During simultaneous pressure and cineangiographic recordings, the jugular venous catheter was slowly withdrawn towards the right atrium, and in the 5th compression cycle (arrow), an abrupt change in pressure contour occurs so that in the latter part of the 5th cycle and during the next two compression cycles, the 'systolic' pressure recorded by the venous catheter equalled the aortic pressure. The site of the pressure transition is demonstrated in Figure 11B (Time lines = 1 s.).

At the nadir of the relaxation phase, forward flow occurs towards and through the right heart, and the pulmonic valve opens widely.

These right heart cineangiographic findings are consistent with radioisotopic studies in dogs performed by Weisfeldt's group, and with Werner's two-dimensional echocardiographic studies in human subjects [22]. Werner's observations demonstrated that the tricuspid valve remained open during compression while the pulmonic valve closed. He noted reflux of contrast medium into the inferior vena cava during compression, and forward flow through the tricuspid valve during relaxation, followed by opening of the pulmonic valve. Further confirmation of the cineangiographic studies of vena caval dynamics was obtained by placing cannulating flow probes in the abdominal vena cava and jugular vein in dogs undergoing CPR (Figure 10). These records reveal major 'systolic' retrograde flow in the inferior vena cava in early systole, with a briefer and lesser magnitude reflux into the jugular vein. During 'diastole', there is forward or positive flow (towards the heart) from both venous tributaries, with a greater net positive flow from the superior tributaries.

4.3. Thoracic inlet valves

Competent venous valves have been shown to be present at the superior thoracic

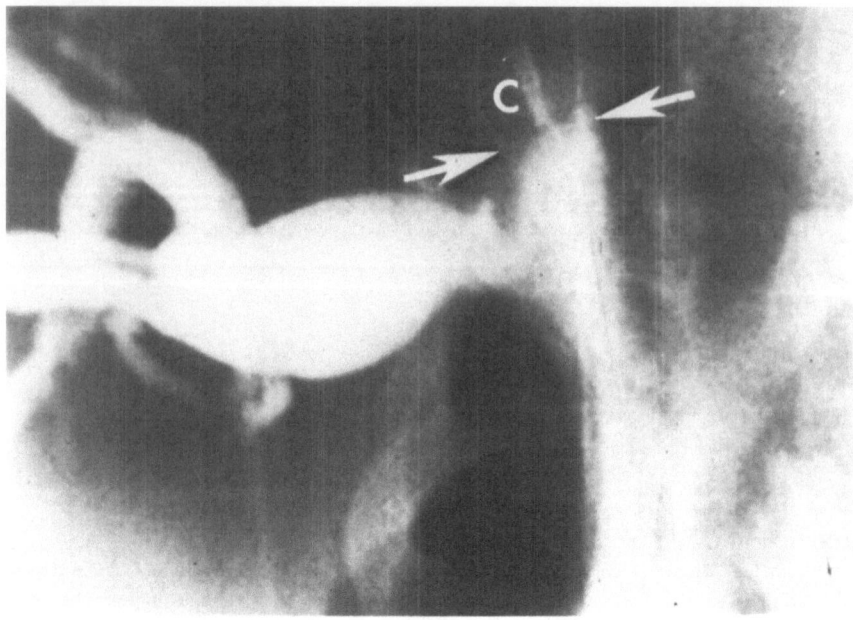

Figure 11B. Angiographic demonstration of thoracic inlet venous valve. An axillary vein injection of contrast medium opacified the junction of the subclavian vein and jugular vein at the apex of the right hemithorax during the catheter withdrawal shown in Figure 11A. With each chest compression, an abrupt horizontal cutoff of refluxing blood into the jugular vein was seen (arrows) and as the micromanometer catheter (C) crossed this site, the pressure transition occurred (Figure 11A).

inlets during CPR. Their function has been demonstrated by means of synchronized cineangiographic pressure recordings [24] (Figure 11). Weisfeldt's group [12] had previously noted the presence of a low jugular venous pressure during CPR compression and had recognized that this low pressure provided the arteriovenous gradient necessary for blood flow, attributing the low pressure to venous collapse. Niemann and coworkers demonstrated that valves at the superior thoracic inlets closed competently during abrupt rises in intrathoracic pressure, as seen in CPR or cough CPR (Figure 12); they provided evidence of specific anatomic sites responsible for the prevention of venous backflow and the creation of a low pressure venous bed.

The presence of these valves at the superior thoracic inlets has been noted in anatomical dissections in man, but their clinical significance has been obscured by the fact that there is usually a faithful transmission of right atrial pressure events into the jugular veins. It appears that the jugular valves close under conditions of abrupt, high pressure rises in the venous or intrathoracic pressure, presumably for the teleologic purpose of preventing high pressure surges into the cerebral venous vascular bed during coughing, retching, or straining.

The paramount importance of these valves during CPR can be inferred from the

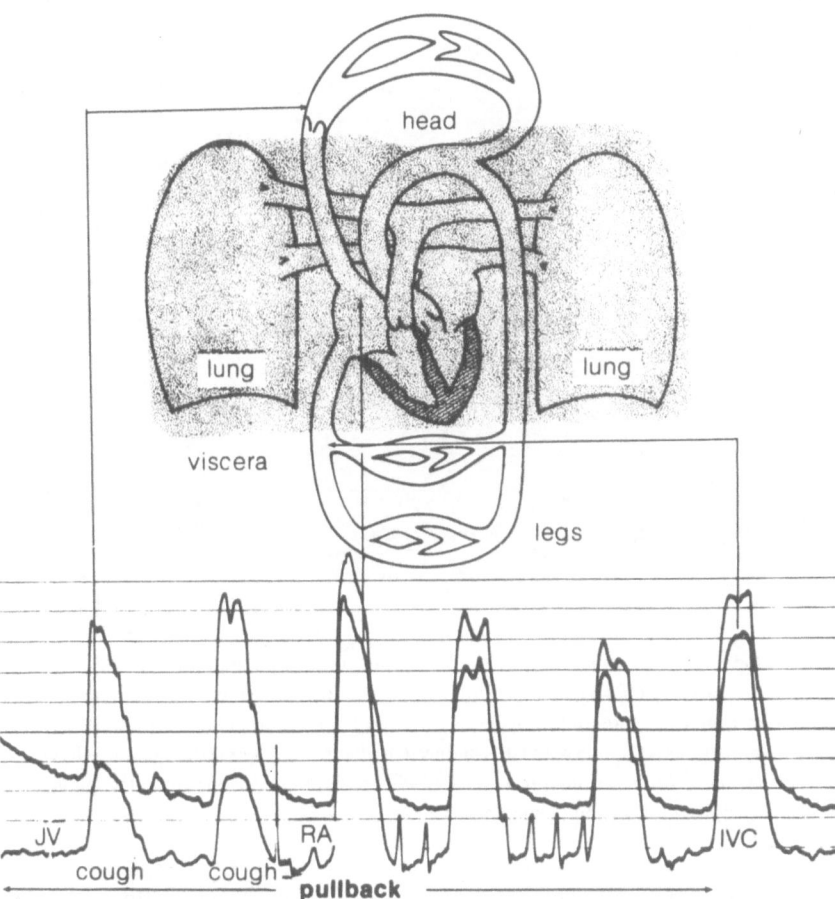

Figure 12. Cough CPR-hemodynamic demonstration of jugular venous valve competence during ventricular fibrillation.

During cough CPR in a dog (Rosborough's technique), a slow withdrawal tracing is obtained from a micromanometer catheter which is initially in the jugular vein (JV) and withdrawn through the right atrium (RA) to the abdominal inferior vena cava (IVC). An equisensitive micromanometer catheter has been placed in the aorta. With each cough, the pressure in the aorta rises to more than 80 mm Hg (pressure lines = 10 mm Hg), while the jugular venous pressure rises to 35–40 mm Hg. As the catheter is withdrawn to the right atrium, large *a* waves are seen between coughs due to continued sinus rhythm in the atrium despite ventricular fibrillation, and pressure rises to nearly aortic level during cough. As the catheter is withdrawn further into the inferior vena cava, the *a* waves are no longer seen, and the phasic pressures continue to approximate aortic pressures during cough. These pressure events result from the global increase in intrathoracic structures. The jugular vein is protected by a venous valve, but the inferior vena cava is not.

fact that they supply 'the missing link' in our understanding of several paradoxes that obscured our knowledge of the mechanism of blood flow during both CPR and cough CPR. As noted above, the first important paradox was the observation that there did not seem to be an arteriovenous pressure gradient during CPR compres-

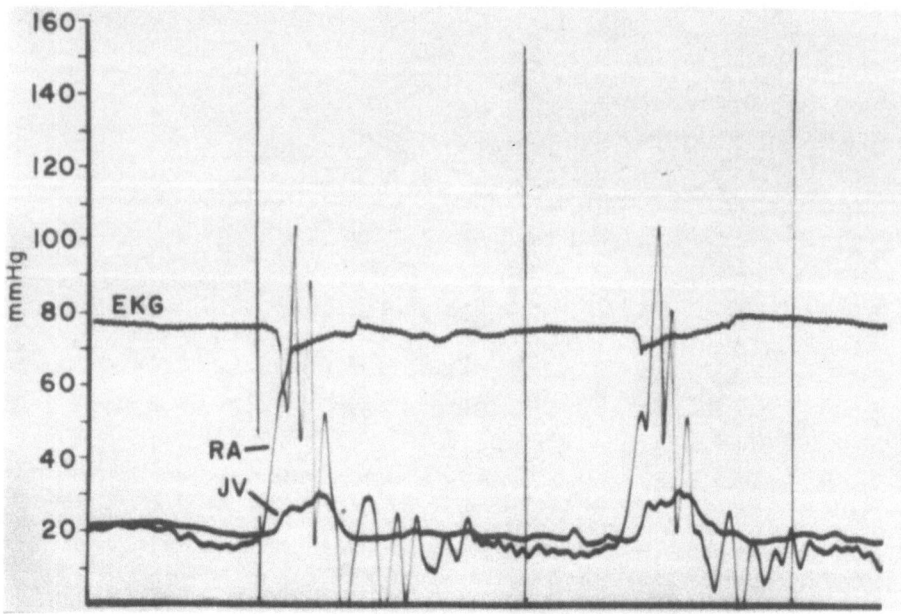

Figure 13. Hemodynamic demonstration of jugular venous function in man during CPR.

Catheters were placed in the right atrium and jugular vein to record equisensitive pressures from the same baseline in a patient who could not be resuscitated from cardiopulmonary arrest. The electrocardiogram demonstrates a flat line with CPR-induced artifacts. The right atrial pressure (RA) rises to a higher level than the jugular venous pressure (JV) with each compression, while the jugular venous pressure is higher during relaxation (Time lines = 1 s.)

sion, and consequently no apparent driving force for blood to flow. Weale and Rothwell-Jackson [9] noted no pressure difference between the iliac artery and vein, and many others had observed that the atrial and aortic pressures rose to the same levels during CPR compression. Since neither of these venous sites is protected by venous valves, it can be understood why they are exposed to the high pressures generated within the chest (and abdomen) during CPR and cough. The low pressure in the brachiocephalic venous bed, protected by the venous valves, provides the explanation not only for flow to this bed, but also for the disproportionately high flow to this vascular bed during CPR and cough. The abdominal vascular bed, unprotected by venous valves, has near-equal arterial and venous pressures which are transmitted through vascular channels and with the increased intra-abdominal pressure generated during CPR and cough CPR, this vascular bed thus receives little or no perfusion during 'systole'. There are valves proximal to the inferior inlets to the abdominal cavity, but we have not studied the dynamics of blood flow to the lower extremities during CPR or cough CPR.

Confirmation of the importance of thoracic inlet venous valve function in man is provided by several clinical observations. Simultaneous pressure recordings from the right atrium and jugular vein during CPR demonstrate that there is a significant pressure difference (Figure 13), and thus a low pressure jugular venous bed during CPR compression in man. Weisfeldt's group has recorded pressure withdrawals from the right atrium to the jugular vein during CPR in man, and observed an abrupt pressure transition as the catheter was pulled from the intrathoracic to the extrathoracic venous bed. Lastly, Weisfeldt's group has recorded cineangiograms and pressure recordings confirming the closure of these thoracic inlet veins during coughing in conscious human subjects.

4.4. The thoracic pump

Since many observations in man and experimental animals not only fail to confirm the presence of a 'cardiac pump' during CPR, but indeed are quite incompatible with such a mechanism, an alternative mechanism for perfusion during CPR must be proposed which is in concert with the objective findings. It is our belief that the 'thoracic pump' mechanism best fits the observed phenomena. Thoracic compression or rises in intrathoracic pressure generated by cough increase the pressure almost uniformly throughout the thorax (and abdomen) and these pressure rises can be recorded faithfully within every intravascular compartment, hollow viscus, or potential space within these compartments, as well as within the airways if the 'leak' to the atmosphere is prevented by clamping of the endotracheal tube (or closing the glottis in cough). This uniform application of pressure throughout the vascular beds contained within these compartments fails to provide any intrathoracic or intra-abdominal arteriovenous pressure gradient, but because of closure of superior thoracic inlet venous valves, a low pressure brachiocephalic venous bed is created. The intrathoracic pressure drives blood through the arteries towards the low pressure venous bed(s).

During relaxation between compressions, there is a small arteriovenous pressure gradient resulting from the higher arterial tonus, which may provide some flow to the coronary and visceral beds. Also during relaxation, there is flow towards and through the right heart, resulting from the buildup of extrathoracic venous pressure during compression, the elastic recoil of the thorax, and the increased compliance of the relatively 'emptied' intrathoracic vascular structures.

One could argue that the 'thoracic pump' terminology is necessarily restrictive, since the abdominal cavity and thoracic cavity are exposed to near-identical pressure fluctuations during CPR and cough CPR. Indeed, preliminary experiments by Rosborough [25] have indicated that abdominal compression CPR may produce greater carotid blood flow than thoracic compression CPR in experimental animals. Nevertheless, we believe that the 'thoracic pump' concept provides a readily understood mechanism which explains better the mechanism of blood flow than does the 'cardiac pump'.

Since the 'cardiac pump' mechanism is widely taught and has provided an explanation for the generation of blood flow during CPR for over 20 years, there is a considerable reluctance to abandon the concept entirely. It is our feeling that we

42

cannot rule out any contribution whatsoever from a 'cardiac pump' in every instance of CPR. Individual variability in thoracic cage anatomy and compliance, size and anatomical location of the heart within the thorax, and differences in technique of application of CPR make it possible that in some circumstances a 'cardiac pump' may be operative. Clearly further observations are needed to clarify this continuing controversy.

5. SOME CAVEATS

Our research team believes that there is a considerable body of evidence from laboratory experiments and clinical observations that supports the 'new' mechanism of blood flow in CPR, and although this new mechanism opens up many new possibilities for improving vital organ blood flow through a more complete understanding of the hemodynamics involved, we feel obligated to urge caution on those who might wish to completely abandon the standard method of performing CPR.

It is important to point out that standard CPR has been directly responsible for the salvage of many thousands of 'hearts too good to die', and that there are many anecdotal instances of CPR-supported circulation for 30 min or more with minimal vital organ ischemic damage. It is therefore clear that CPR works. The new concepts of CPR and the proposed mechanisms for improving it should be scrutinized closely as should any therapeutic modality which is compared to an established treatment. The benefits of changing the technique should be weighed against any possible risks. For example, several groups have demonstrated an improved arterial pressure and carotid blood flow to accompany simultaneous inflation and compression, or 'new' CPR. Are there any risks associated with this seemingly innocuous modification? There are obvious potential hazards such as barotrauma due to high pressure airway inflation, gastric insufflation if the technique is carried out without a cuffed endotracheal tube, and inhibition of venous return if inflation is not precisely synchronized with compression.

It has been shown that abdominal binding and negative 'diastolic' airway pressure can increase carotid artery flow, but these techniques are not without hazard if performed without appreciation of potential hepatic laceration, and it requires considerable complexity to achieve negative phasic airway pressure synchronized with diastole.

6. FUTURE CONSIDERATIONS

The new concepts of the mechanism of blood flow provide considerable promise for improvements in vital organ perfusion, not only during CPR, but also in methods of circulatory assistance of the compromised heart. We believe that the future is bright for research into the mechanisms of improving and expanding the usefulness of a technique that has served mankind well for over twenty years.

ACKNOWLEDGEMENTS

This work was funded in part by Investigative Group Award 427IG11 American Heart Association, Greater Los Angeles Affiliate and by a grant from Physio-Control Corporation, Seattle, WA, U.S.A.

REFERENCES

1. Lown B, Wolf M: Approaches to sudden death from coronary heart disease. Circulation 44:130–142, 1971.
2. Guerci A: Sudden death – Medical Staff Conference, Univ. of Calif., San Francisco. West J Med 133:313, 1980.
3. Kuller L, Lilienfeld A, Fisher R: Epidemiological study of sudden and unexpected deaths due to arteriosclerotic heart disease. Circulation 34:1056–1068, 1966.
4. Thompson RG, Hallstrom AP, Cobb LA: Bystander-initiated cardiopulmonary resuscitation in the management of ventricular fibrillation. Ann Int Med 90:737–740, 1979.
5. Overbeck W: Historical views concerning cardiac arrest and resuscitation. In: Cardiac Arrest and Resuscitation. (Stephenson HE Jr, ed.) 3rd Edn, pp. 26–40. The C.V. Mosby Company, St. Louis, 1969.
6. Stephenson HE Jr: Artificial maintenance of circulation: open-chest resuscitation. In: Cardiac Arrest and Resuscitation. (Stephenson HE Jr, ed.) 3rd edn, pp. 211–231. The C.V. Mosby Company, St. Louis, 1969.
7. Kouwenhoven WB, Jude JR, Knickerbocker GG: Closed chest cardiac massage. JAMA 173:1064–1067, 1960.
8. Bahnson HT: The present status of closed-chest cardiac massage. Surgical Rounds, p. 55, July 1980.
9. Weale FE, Rothwell-Jackson RL: The efficiency of cardiac massage. Lancet 1:990–992, 1962.
10. MacKenzie GJ, Taylor SH, MacDonald AH, Donald KW: Hemodynamic effects of external cardiac compression. Lancet 1:1342–1345, 1964.
11. Thomsen JE, Stenlund RR, Rowe GG: Intracardiac pressures during closed-chest cardiac massage. JAMA 205:116–118, 1968.
12. Rudikoff MT, Maughan WL, Effron M, Freund P, Weisfeldt ML: Mechanisms of blood flow during cardiopulmonary resuscitation. Circulation 61:345–352, 1980.
13. Criley JM: CPR and emergency cardiac care, looking to the future. In: Proceedings of New York Heart Association Conference on Current Practice and Current Research in Cardiopulmonary Resuscitation and Emergency Cardiac Care. (Schluger J, Lyon AF, eds.) p. 47, E.M. Books, 1980.
14. Sones FM Jr: Cine coronary arteriography. In: The Heart. (Hurst JW, Logue RB, eds.), pp. 377–385. New York: McGraw-Hill, 1970.
15. King SB III, Douglas JS: Coronary arteriography and left ventriculography. In: The Heart, Arteries and Veins. (Hurst JW, Logue RB, Schlant RC, Wenger NK, eds.). 4th Edn, p. 401. New York: McGraw-Hill, 1978.
16. Criley JM, Blaufuss AH, Kissel GL: Cough-induced cardiac compression, self-administered form of cardiopulmonary resuscitation. JAMA 236:1246–1250, 1976.
17. Blaufuss AH, Brown DC, Jackson B, Criley JM: Does coughing produce cardiac output during cardiac arrest? Circulation 55–56: (Suppl III):68, 1977 (Abstract).
18. Niemann JT, Rosborough J, Hausknecht M, Brown D, Criley JM: Cough-CPR, Documentation of systemic perfusion in man and in an experimental model: a 'window' to the mechanism of blood flow in external CPR. Crit Care Med 8:141–146, 1980.
19. Ross BB, Gramiak R, Rahn H: Physical dynamics of the cough mechanism. J Appl Physiol 8: 264–268, 1955.

44

20. Giuntini C, Lewis ML, Luis AS, Harvey RM: A study of the pulmonary blood volume in man by quantitative radiocardiography. J Clin Invest 42:1589–1605, 1963.
21. Rosborough JP, Niemann JT, Criley JM: Unpublished observations.
22. Werner JA, Green HL, Janko C, Cobb LA: Visualization of cardiac valve motion in man during external chest compression using two-dimensional echocardiography. Implications regarding the mechanism of blood flow. Circulation 63:1417–1421, 1981.
23. Niemann JT, Rosborough J, Hausknecht M, Criley JM: The effects of lung inflation on right heart flow in CPR. Circulation 62 (Suppl III):133, 1980 (Abstract).
24. Niemann JT, Rosborough J, Hausknecht M, Garner D, Criley JM: Pressure-synchronized cine-angiographic observations during experimental cardiopulmonary resuscitation. Circulation 64: 985–991, 1981.
25. Rosborough JP, Niemann JT, Criley JM, O'Bannon W: Lower abdominal compression with synchronized ventilation: a CPR modality. Circulation 64 (Part II): 303, 1981 (Abstract).

3. ETIOLOGY OF VENTRICULAR ARRHYTHMIAS IN THE EARLY PHASE OF MYOCARDIAL ISCHEMIA

RE-ENTRY, FOCUS AND ACTION OF DRUGS

MICHIEL J. JANSE

Since the work of Harris and coworkers it has been common knowledge that ventricular arrhythmias after coronary artery occlusion in animal experiments occur in two distinct phases [1, 2]. The first one corresponding to the acute phase of ischemia, will last until 15–30 min after coronary occlusion, the second phase will start after 4–8 h and last for 24–48 h. Exact figures of the incidence of ventricular arrhythmias in the early phase are sparse, but in a large series of 351 dogs in which complete occlusion of a major coronary artery was performed, ventricular fibrillation occurred in 28% of the animals in the first 30 min [3]. Our own experience with isolated perfused hearts of pigs and dogs, driven at a constant rate just above the sinus rate, in which the left anterior descending artery was occluded, indicates that ventricular premature beats occur in 72% of cases, ventricular tachycardia (more than five consecutive ectopic beats) in 45% and ventricular fibrillation in 32% of cases, all within 2–8 min after occlusion [4]. It is not known whether a bimodal distribution of ventricular arrhythmias in myocardial infarction in man exists, but the early arrhythmia phase in the animal model may be related to the 'prehospital' phase of arrhythmias in human infarction. The incidence of ventricular arrhythmias in the first hours of myocardial infarction in man varies widely in different reports, but figures approximating 70% for ventricular premature beats, 40% for ventricular tachycardia, and 30% for ventricular fibrillation have been reported [5, 6].

The purpose of this paper is to describe, firstly, the electrophysiological changes that occur in the first 15 min after coronary occlusion. Secondly, mapping experiments will be described, which allowed for the identification of patterns of excitation during spontaneous arrhythmias and the demonstration of circus movement re-entry in ventricular tachycardia and fibrillation. At the same time, these experiments provided evidence that the ectopic beats which initiate both ventricular tachycardia and fibrillation are caused by a mechanism other than circus movement re-entry; various possibilities including the role of injury currents will be discussed. Finally, the effect of certain drugs on the electrical changes during ischemia, and their consequent antiarrhythmic effects will be shown.

Adgey, AAJ (ed): Acute phase of ischemic heart disease and myocardial infarction.
© *1982, Martinus Nijhoff, The Hague, Boston, London. ISBN-13: 978-94-009-7581-1*

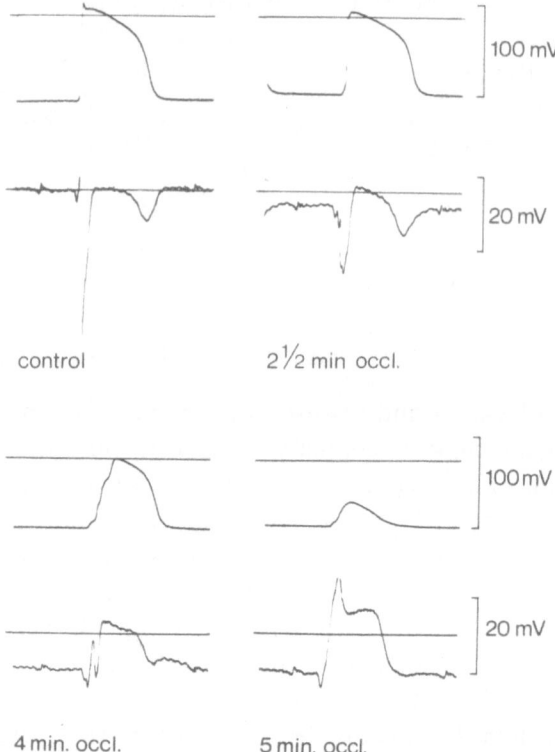

Figure 1. Electrophysiological changes in the first minutes after coronary artery occlusion. Transmembrane potentials (upper tracings) and local DC-extracellular electrogram (lower tracings) recorded from the left ventricular subepicardium before and after occlusion of the left anterior descending coronary artery in an isolated perfused porcine heart. Horizontal lines are zero potential levels. Note the decrease in resting membrane potential and the corresponding depression of the TQ-segment in the extracellular potential ($2\frac{1}{2}$ min after occlusion). Later, action potential amplitude and upstroke velocity decrease and true ST-elevation develops. (Reproduced with permission from M.J. Janse and D. Durrer. In: Experimental Ischemia and Infarction. (W. Schaper, ed.) New York: Marcel Dekker, 1981).

1. ELECTROPHYSIOLOGIC CHANGES DURING ACUTE REGIONAL ISCHEMIA

In Figure 1, the changes in transmembrane potential and in the corresponding local DC extracellular electrogram that occur in ventricular myocardium after coronary artery occlusion are shown. The recordings were made from an isolated porcine heart, perfused with a 1:1 mixture of blood and modified Tyrode solution according to the Langendorff technique. Flexibly mounted microelectrodes (one intracellularly, the other as closely as possible in the extracellular space) recorded the transmembrane potential. At the same site, a cotton wick electrode recorded the DC extracellular potential with respect to the DC potential of the aortic root.

The first change that occurs after occlusion of the left anterior descending co-

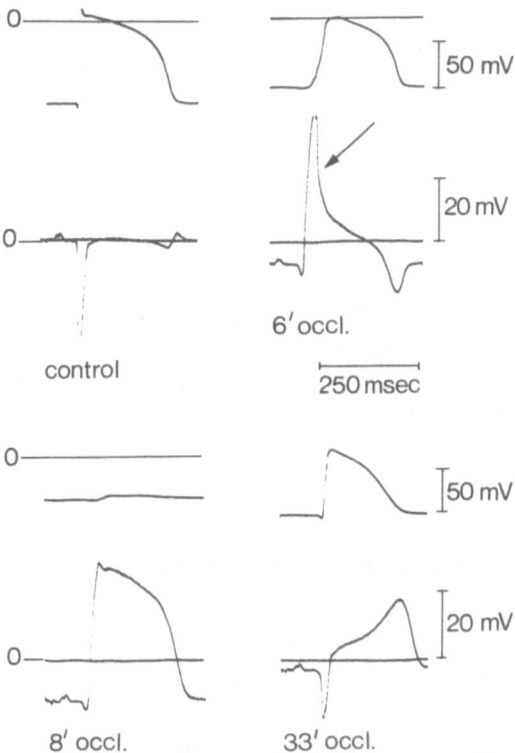

control   6' occl.

250 msec

8' occl.   33' occl.

Figure 2. Transmembrane potentials and local DC electrograms from the left ventricular subepicardium of an isolated porcine heart. After 6 min of ischemia, action potential upstroke is slow and activation of the ischemic cell is delayed (arrow points to late intrinsic deflection in the extracellular complex). Note the disappearance of transmembrane action potential after 8 min (extracellular complex is then monophasic) and reappearance of electrical activity at 33 min. (Reproduced with permission from M.J. Janse and D. Durrer, Ned. Tijdschr. Geneesk. 122, 1737–1741, 1978.)

ronary artery is a decrease in resting membrane potential. In the example shown, resting membrane potential decreased from a control value of − 96 mV to − 86mV within 2.5 min after occlusion. By that time, action potential configuration had hardly changed. The loss in resting membrane potential is reflected in the extracellular electrogram by depression of the TQ segment. If extracellular potentials had been recorded via metal electrodes and AC amplifiers such as standard electrocardiographs, the TQ segment depression would have been recorded as an elevation of the ST segment. Only the use of a DC recording system enables one to distinguish between negative and positive extracellular potential changes.

After 4 min of occlusion, resting membrane potential decreased further to − 75 mV, and the depression of the TQ segment changed from − 2 to − 11 mV. By then the upstroke of the action potential had become slower, its amplitude was diminished and the moment of activation of the ischemic cell was delayed. After 5 min, the action potential was reduced to a small amplitude response of which it is doubtful

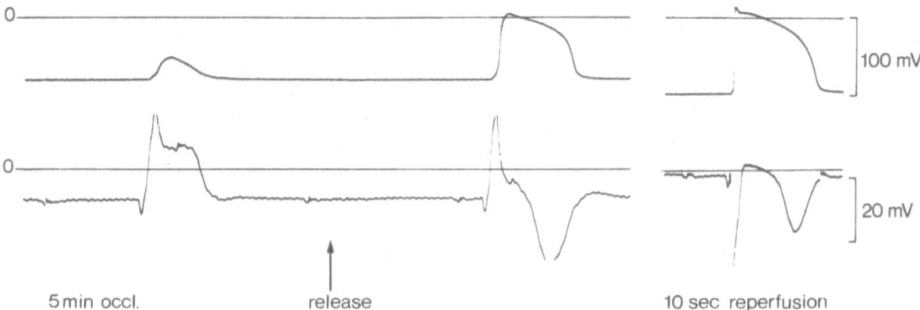

Figure 3. Reversibility of electrical changes during ischemia. Clamp on the left anterior descending artery was released after 5 min of occlusion. Action potentials appear immediately without change in resting potential. After 10 sec, action potentials are completely normal. (Reproduced with permission from M.J. Janse and D. Durrer, In: Experimental Ischemia and Infarction, (W. Schaper, ed. New York: Marcel Dekker, 1981.)

whether it is able to propagate. In the extracellular electrogram true ST elevation is now apparent. (In the isolated pig heart, TQ segment depression begins on the average 1.5 min after coronary artery occlusion, true ST elevation after 4 min. In working hearts in situ these changes occur earlier, and TQ depression may become apparent already after 30 s.)

With occlusion maintained, the membrane depolarizes further, until at resting membrane potential levels of -60 to -65 mV no action potential can be elicited by activity propagating from the nonischemic myocardium. This happens between 5 and 10 min. The accompanying extracellular complex is completely monophasic, displaying a TQ segment depression of about -15 mV, and a ST segment elevation of about $+25$ mV. This phase of unresponsiveness, as shown in Figure 2, the data of which taken from another experiment, is transient. With coronary occlusion maintained, excitability returns to previously inexcitable cells after 20–40 min. The action potentials are abnormal in that they have a short duration and a reduced amplitude and upstroke velocity, yet they are able to propagate. After about one hour of occlusion, the ischemic cells become inexcitable again, and this time for good.

The changes described here are in agreement with findings by other authors using different techniques. Extracellular epicardial recording showed that during the first minutes following coronary artery occlusion, epicardial potentials were delayed and fragmented, whereas after 15–20 min the delay had disappeared and near-normal activation times were found [7, 8]. The reasons for the temporal 'improvement' of electrical activity are unclear as yet.

Depending on the duration of the period of ischemia these dramatic alterations in the electrical activity are reversible upon reperfusion. Figure 3 shows the almost immediate recovery of electrical activity when after 5 min of occlusion reperfusion is allowed by releasing the clamp on the left anterior descending artery. It is of interest to note that resting potential level does not change immediately and that at the same level of resting membrane potential a very small response is present during occlusion, whereas a large amplitude response, albeit with a slow upstroke, occurs immediately upon reperfusion. Within 10 s resting membrane potential returned to the control level and action potential regained its original configuration.

1.1. The decrease in resting membrane potential

It has long been known that myocardial cells release potassium during acute ischemia [9] and that, also as a consequence of the lack of flow, potassium ions accumulate in the extracellular space. Recently, the extracellular K^+ activity has been measured directly by means of potassium sensitive electrodes inserted into the ventricular wall of porcine hearts [10, 11]. An increase in extracellular K^+ activity was already apparent 15 s after coronary artery occlusion, and after 5–8 min extracellular K^+ concentrations had risen to levels between 10 and 14 mM. It is not clear whether the loss of potassium ions from ischemic cells is primarily due to either an inhibition of the Na^+/K^+ pump caused by lack of oxygen, or to an anoxia-induced increased K^+ conductance of the cell membrane [12]. It is reasonable to suppose that the partial depolarization of ischemic cells occurring at the same time as the rise in extracellular potassium concentration, is primarily caused by the changed gradient for K^+ across the cell membrane.

1.2. Changes in action potential upstroke characteristics

Action potential amplitude and upstroke velocity are dependent on the level of the resting membrane potential [13]. At first glance it would be reasonable to postulate that the decrease in action potential amplitude, and the decrease in dV/dt max are secondary to the decrease in resting membrane potential. Several observations, however, suggest that the partial inactivation of the rapid sodium inward current by depolarization of the resting membrane potential is not sufficient to account for the marked depression of action potential upstroke characteristics seen during ischemia. When the left anterior descending coronary artery in isolated bloodperfused pig hearts is selectively perfused with solutions containing high K^+ levels, transmembrane action potentials recorded from the area perfused by the left anterior descending coronary artery have larger amplitudes and show faster upstrokes than action potentials recorded from the same sites during occlusion of the same artery [14]. The potassium levels of the solutions used to perfuse the left anterior descending coronary artery were in the range of 10–14 mM, which were the levels measured in the experiments of Hill and Gettes [10] and Hirche et al. [11] in the in situ porcine heart. Hill and Gettes [10] found that activation delay was more pronounced during ischemia at a certain extracellular K^+ level than during regional perfusion of the coronary artery in the same heart with solutions containing the same potassium concentration.

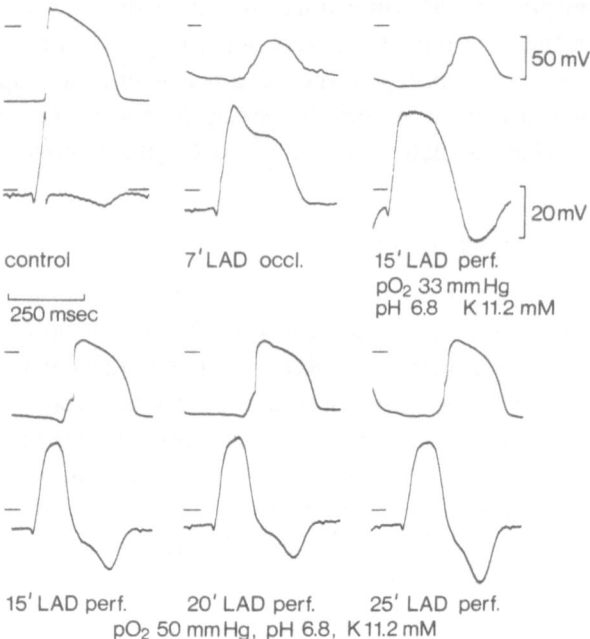

Figure 4. Comparison of the effects of regional ischemia, hypoxia and hyperkalemia on intra- and extracellular potentials in the intact porcine heart. Upper tracings: transmembrane potentials, lower tracings: local DC extracellular electrogram. All recordings were made at the same site, in the subepi-cardium of that part of the left ventricle perfused by the left anterior descending artery (LAD). Recordings were made under control conditions, 7 min following occlusion of the LAD, and 15 min after perfusing the LAD selectively with a hypoxic, glucose-free, acidotic and hyperkalemic solution (upper panel). Note similarity in potentials during LAD occlusion and LAD perfusion. In lower panel, after a suitably normal reperfusion period, the LAD was again perfused with the acidotic high K^+ solution, but PO_2 was increased from 33 to 50 mmHg. Potentials are now far less depressed. (Reproduced with permission from M.J. Janse, H. Moréna, J. Cinca, J.W.T. Fiolet, W.J. Krieger, D. Durrer, J. Physiol. (Paris) 76, 785–790, 1980.)

In our experiments [14] the configuration of transmembrane action potentials recorded during ischemia could be obtained neither by regional perfusion with high K^+ solutions nor by solutions made hypoxic (pO_2 of 7–10 mmHg) and containing no glucose. However, as shown in Figure 4, when the left anterior descending coronary artery was perfused with a hypoxic, acidotic solution containing a high K^+ level, the recorded action potentials were very similar in appearance to those recorded during occlusion of the same artery. Apparently, the combination of lack of oxygen and substrate and lack of washout (high extracellular potassium, low pH) has an extra depressant effect on the ionic mechanisms responsible for the gene-ration of the action potential upstroke.

Information about the ionic nature of the currents generating the depressed upstroke during ischemia can only be obtained via indirect means. There has been some speculation whether the action potential upstroke in ischemia is caused by a

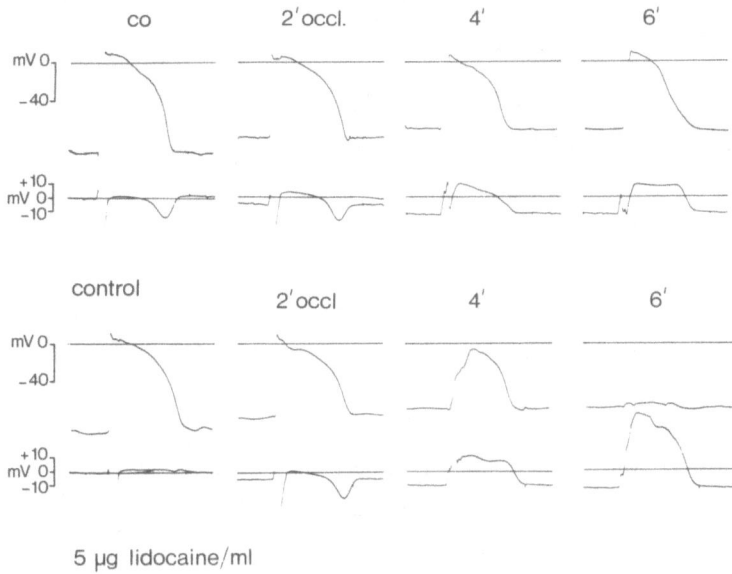

Figure 5. Effect of lidocaine on intra- and extracellular potential changes induced by ischemia. When lidocaine is administered prior to coronary artery occlusion, the depression of action potential characteristics is accelerated. Within 6 min, the cell recorded from is inexcitable in the presence of lidocaine, whereas in its absence a sizeable action potential is still recorded at that time in a previous occlusion. (Reproduced with permission from M.J. Janse and D. Durrer, In: Experimental Ischemia and Infarction. (W. Schaper, ed.) New York: Marcel Dekker, 1981).

depressed fast inward current, carried by Na^+ ions, or by a true slow inward current, carried by Ca^{++} and Na^+ ions, in the presence of a totally inactivated fast inward current. The distinction between the two possibilities is of more than academic interest since fast and slow inward currents are affected by different classes of anti-arrhythmic drugs. One way to investigate the contributions of fast and slow inward currents in the generation of the action potential is to study the effects of different blocking agents.

From studies on isolated Purkinje fibers it is known that lidocaine depressed the fast inward current, but has little effect on slow calcium responses [15]. Verapamil, on the other hand, is a potent blocker of the slow inward current. In Figure 5, the effects of lidocaine on intra- and extracellular potentials during ischemia are shown. When repeated coronary artery occlusions are performed in isolated hearts for periods of 10–15 min, reperfusion leads to a rapid normalization of electrical activity. However, the electrophysiological changes during first and second occlusions differ; those during second, third and fourth occlusions are the same [16]. In studies concerning the effects of drugs in acute ischemia, in which each heart serves as its own control, the first two occlusions must be performed in the absence of a drug. The second occlusion is the control occlusion, and drugs can be added prior to the third and fourth occlusions. Figure 5 shows that lidocaine, administered before

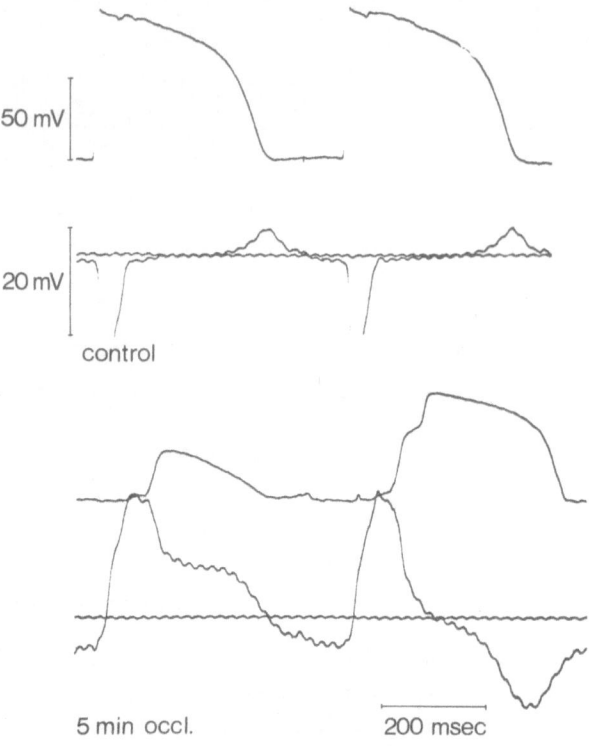

50 mV

20 mV

control

5 min occl.   200 msec

Figure 6. Alternation in action potential amplitude and duration 5 min after coronary occlusion (bottom) (top: control recordings). Note separation of action potential upstroke into two components (last potential in lower row). The first component might be caused by the depressed fast inward current which brings the potential into the range where the slow inward current is activated, which might be responsible for the second component. Delayed repolarization of the ischemic cell leads to negative T wave in local electrogram. (Reproduced with permission from [18].)

the third occlusion, accelerates and exaggerates the depression of the action potential during ischemia. Whereas, in the absence of the drug, a sizeable action potential is still present after 6 min of occlusion, the cell has become irresponsive in the presence of lidocaine.

Extensive mapping studies showed that at comparable times following coronary artery occlusion, the number of inexcitable sites was greater in the presence of lidocaine [16]. Lidocaine had no effect on the time course of change in resting membrane potential during ischemia. Thus, at similar resting membrane potential levels, lidocaine had an extra depressant effect on action potential upstroke characteristics. These findings are in agreement with the results of Lazzara et al. [17] who showed that action potentials recorded from excised hearts 1–3 days after coronary ligation could be abolished by adding lidocaine. These findings, together with the observation that in isolated hearts ischemic cells show no response when the membrane potential is depolarized to a level around -60 mV, at which level the fast

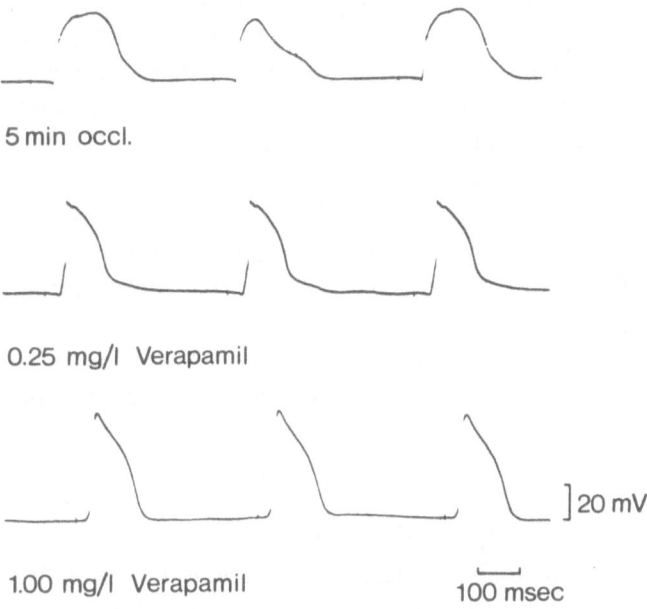

5 min occl.

0.25 mg/l Verapamil

] 20 mV

1.00 mg/l Verapamil   ⌐ 100 msec

Figure 7. Effects of verapamil on transmembrane potentials recorded after 5 min of ischemia in different occlusions in the same heart. Verapamil abolishes the alternation present in the control occlusion, and improves action potential upstroke characteristics. (Unpublished results of M.J. Janse, A. Wilde, I. Kodama.)

sodium inward current is totally inactivated, can be taken to indicate that the action potential in the very early phase of ischemia, as well as in the late phase (several days after coronary occlusion) of infarction, is a 'depressed fast response'.

What, then, is the effect of ischemia on the slow inward current? Very frequently during the first minutes of coronary occlusion the ischemic cells display an alternation in action potential amplitude and duration, and the upstroke of the action potential having the large amplitude is often clearly separated into two compartments (see Figure 6) [18–20]. Similar action potentials were found by Mascher [21] in canine ventricular myocardium exposed to critically elevated potassium levels. He demonstrated that the first component was due to the, depressed, fast sodium inward current which brought the membrane potential into the range where the slow inward current became activated, which was responsible for the second phase of the upstroke and determined the duration of the plateau. The alternation, which is so characteristic for the early phase of ischemia, could be due to activation of the slow inward current only during every second beat. If so, this would indicate that the slow inward current is depressed by ischemia even more rapidly than the fast inward current [22].

In Figure 7 the effects of verapamil on ischemic action potentials are shown. During the occlusions performed in the absence of the drug, alternation was clearly present. Verapamil abolished the alternation. In the presence of verapamil action potentials were much shorter, showed no plateau, and the upstroke had only one component. At similar moments after coronary occlusion, depolarization of the resting membrane potential was less, and action potential upstroke was faster in the presence of verapamil. The reasons for this are not certain. It is possible that because of the marked negative inotropic effect of verapamil in the dosage used, energy depletion was less during ischemia, and K^+ accumulation in the extracellular space might have been reduced. Also, it is possible that the reduction in intracellular Ca^{++} concentration due to verapamil might have prevented an increase in K^+ conductance [23] and consequently have prevented to some degree the loss of K^+ from the ischemic cells.

The experiments described above strongly suggest that ischemia depressed both the fast and the slow inward currents, and that the depressed action potentials in the acute phase are 'depressed fast responses'.

1.3. Recovery of excitability

Because the action potential of ischemic cells shortens it is generally assumed that refractory periods shorten as well and, indeed, many authors who measured refractory periods with electrical stimuli reported on short refractory periods in ischemic myocardium [24]. As pointed out by Lazzara et al. [25] there are several ways in which refractoriness can be defined. Firstly by applying electrical stimuli of fixed strength at varying coupling intervals and determining the shortest interval at which a response can be elicited. Secondly, the nature of the elicited response can be taken into account: it has long been known that in partially depolarized cells graded responses can be elicited after full repolarization has occurred [26–28]. The refractory period can then be defined as the shortest interval at which a response, even when it is a very low amplitude action potential with a slow upstroke, can be obtained, or the interval after which full recovery of excitability has occurred, and the responses are the same as those elicited at the basic heart rate. In acutely ischemic cells, the phenomenon of postrepolarization refractoriness actually prolongs the refractory period thus defined despite shortening of the transmembrane action potential [19, 25].

It is known [28] that at critically reduced resting membrane potentials, the recovery from inactivation of both fast and slow inward currents is markedly delayed, and that full recovery of excitability outlasts complete repolarization. The dependence of recovery of excitability in partially depolarized ischemic myocardium is one of the most important determinants for the occurrence of slow conduction and conduction block, both being necessary requirements for re-entry. Differences of only a few millivolts in resting potential of adjacent groups of cells may lead to a marked spatial disparity in refractoriness. At a certain coupling interval the least depolarized cell group may exhibit an action potential with a low upstroke velocity, which will propagate slowly, whereas the cells with a slightly lower resting membrane potential are at that time inexcitable, and there conduction

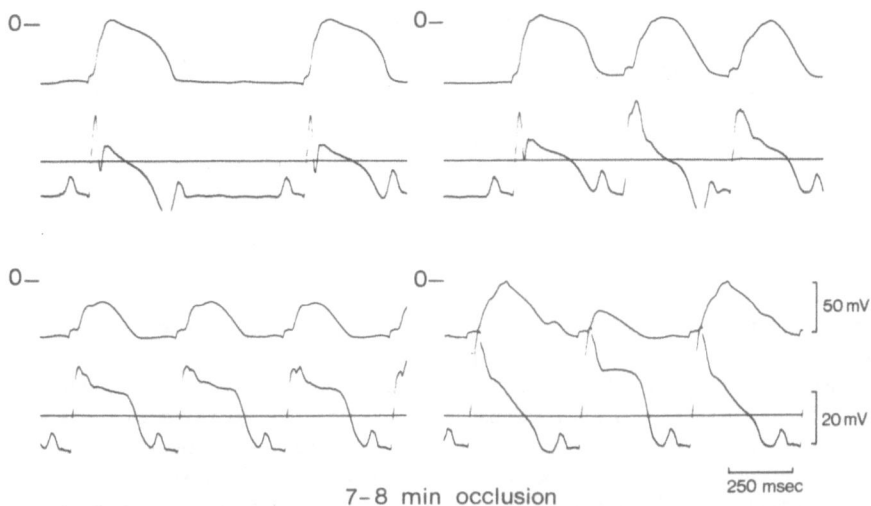

0—

0—

50 mV

20 mV

7– 8 min occlusion

250 msec

Figure 8. Effects of an increase in heart rate 7–8 min after occlusion. In the upper left panel there was 2:1 AV block, which in the upper right panel suddenly was transformed into 1:1 AV conduction so that ventricular rate doubled. The lower two panels were recorded 10 and 20 sec later. Note small action potentials in lower left panel and alternation in lower right panel. (Reproduced with permission from M.J. Janse et al. In: Management of ventricular tachycardia, role of mexiletine. (E. Sandoe, D.G. Julian, J.W. Bell eds.) pp. 183–196.) Amsterdam: Excerpta Medica, 1978.

block will occur. The time dependence of recovery of excitability also explains the effects of heart rate on ischemic cells. Whereas in normal myocardium refractory periods shorten when heart rate is increased, in ischemic myocardium the opposite occurs. Cells which at long cycle lengths show large amplitude action potentials, will at short cycle lengths exhibit small amplitude responses of short duration, or 2:1 alternation, such as shown in Figure 8. In the upper right panel, heart rate was suddenly doubled, because the 2:1 AV block present in the upper left panel was abolished (the first action potential is the last one at the slower rate). The two lower panels were recorded 10–20 s later; as a consequence of post-repolarization refractoriness every second action potential is only a very small response (lower right panel), of which it is doubtful whether it is able to propagate.

2. PATTERNS OF ACTIVATION DURING SPONTANEOUS VENTRICULAR ARRHYTHMIAS

By using multiple DC-electrodes, an A/D converter and a computer, 60 extracellular DC electrograms could be recorded simultaneously for periods of 2 s. Signals recorded during the occurrence of single premature beats, ventricular tachycardia and ventricular fibrillation, were stored in the computer and could later be analyzed [4, 29]. In this way isochronic maps could be constructed depicting the pattern of

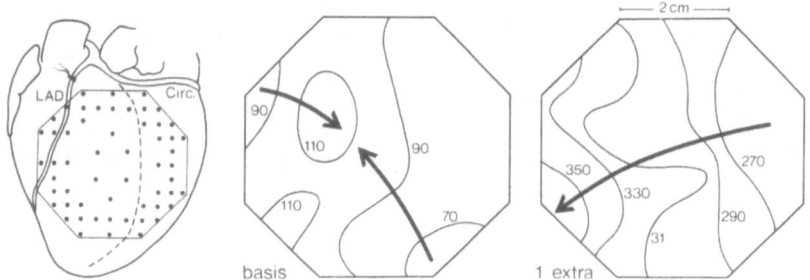

Figure 9. Patterns of activation during a propagated beat from the atrium (basic beat) and the first ectopic beat (1 extra) which induced ventricular tachycardia (Figure 10) which finally degenerated into ventricular fibrillation (Figure 11), 5 min after coronary artery occlusion. On the left, the position of the multiple electrode in the heart is shown schematically. Each dot is an individual electrode terminal. The dotted line indicates the ischemic border. DC extracellular electrograms were simultaneously recorded from 60 terminals for recording periods of 2 s. In the isochronic maps, isochrones separate areas activated within the same 20 ms interval (time zero was the P wave of the basic beat, numbers indicate ms). Note the gap between latest activity during basic beat and earliest ectopic activity, which is found on the non ischemic side of the border.

activation of the area covered by the electrode during the various arrhythmias.

In Figure 9 the left panel shows the configuration of the multiple electrode, each dot indicating an electrode terminal. In this experiment the left anterior descending coronary artery (LAD) was occluded. The dotted line marks the position of the electrophysiological border zone, defined as the area where the TQ-segments of normally propagated beats becomes negative (in other words, it marks the border between tissue with normal resting potentials and tissue with partially depolarized cells). It should be noted that electrodes were present on both sides of the border. The middle panel shows the activation pattern of a basic beat, propagated from the atrium, 4 min after the LAD had been occluded. Isochrones separate areas activated within the same 20 ms interval. Time zero was the P wave and numbers indicate moments of activation in ms. The ischemic area is invaded from two sides, and activation of the area under the electrode takes more than 40 ms (in the control situation, before occlusion, it took 12 ms). In the right panel, the activation pattern of the first ectopic beat, leading to a bout of ventricular tachycardia, is shown. Characteristically, earliest activity was recorded in the non-ischemic myocardium adjacent to the electrophysiological border zone, and no signs of re-entrant activity bridging the gap between latent activity during the basic beat (110 ms) and earliest ectopic activity (270 ms after the P wave of the basic beat) were found.

In Figure 10 the activation patterns during three consecutive beats of the ventricular tachycardia are shown, which in this instance were the 27th, 28th and 29th ectopic activations of the tachycardia. Time zero was arbitrarily chosen. It can be seen that a circus movement is responsible for the continuation of the arrhythmia; in the first beat, activity circles around a small area of conduction block (the shaded area in the Figure), and completes a full circle in 200 ms. Activity ending at 220 ms,

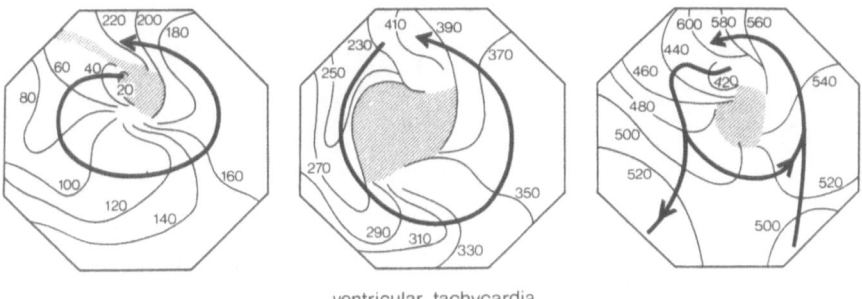

ventricular tachycardia

Figure 10. Activation pattern during ventricular tachycardia. Time zero was arbitrarily chosen. Areas of conduction block are shaded. The tachycardia is sustained by one large circus movement, circling around a zone of temporarily inexcitable ischemic myocardium. Position and dimension of the circus movement change from beat to beat.

continues in the next beat at 230 ms, and again a circus movement, which now has a larger diameter, is completed, but at a shorter revolution time of 180 ms. The circus movement in the third beat has a different position and a smaller diameter, and is joined by another wavefront of unknown origin, emerging at the lower right corner of the electrode at 500 ms.

In Figure 11 the activation pattern of ventricular fibrillation is shown. In contrast to the single, large circus movement present during ventricular tachycardia, the re-entrant wavefronts have now fragmented into multiple wavelets, travelling along tortuous routes among islets of temporarily inexcitable tissue. Sometimes wavefronts join and summate, sometimes they collide and extinguish each other, and only seldom is a small circus movement completed, as is shown in the middle panel in the upper right corner. In general, the pattern bears a striking resemblance to the pattern of fibrillation in the computer model of Moe [30].

The results of our mapping experiments can be summarized as follows. Macro re-entry, in which basically one wavefront circles around an area of temporarily inexcitable tissue within the ischemic myocardium, is responsible for ventricular tachycardia. Such a single circus movement can terminate spontaneously when the excitatory efficacy of the circulating activity is not enough to excite the tissue in the pathway ahead, and sinus rhythm can be restored. However, when the single circus movement breaks up into multiple re-entrant wavelets, and fibrillation ensues, spontaneous termination of the arrhythmia will not occur. Whenever a single wavefront dies out, or two colliding wavefronts extinguish themselves, there are always other wavefronts which will continue to travel around areas of conduction block.

Apparently, re-entry plays a dominant role in tachycardia and fibrillation. However, the ectopic beats which initiate these arrhythmias, appear to have a different genesis. Our experimental findings concerning the genesis of ventricular premature beats during the first minutes of myocardial ischemia (whether single premature

58

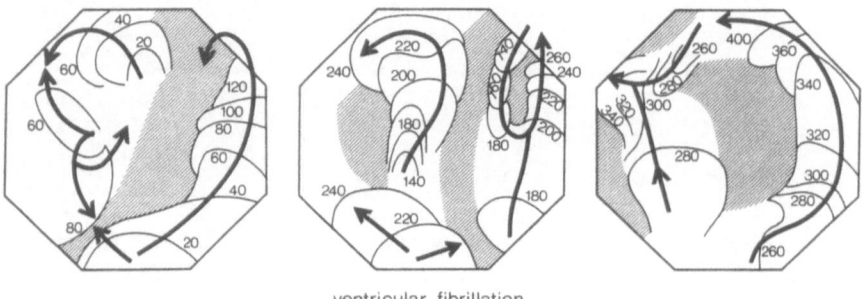

ventricular fibrillation

Figure 11. Activation pattern during ventricular fibrillation. The single circus movement during the tachycardia phase has now fragmented into multiple re-entrant wavelets travelling along tortuous routes between islands of temporarily inexcitable cells. Circus movements are seldom completed. When they are (middle panel), their diameter is small (about 0.5 cm). Collision and fusion of different wavelets frequently occur. (Figures 9, 10 and 11 are modified from [4] and are reproduced with permission.)

beats, multiple premature beats or the initial beats of what finally becomes tachycardia or fibrillation) are the following:

1) In all instances, in both dog and pig hearts, where the activation pattern was mapped, earliest ectopic activity originated in the normal tissue adjacent to the border zone.

2) No evidence was found for re-entrant activity bridging the gap between latest activity during a normally propagated basic beat and earliest activity of the first ectopic beat.

3) Whenever Purkinje activity was recorded from subendocardially located electrodes, it preceded myocardial activity in the ectopic beats.

4) In the majority of the cases (in 21 out of 30 hearts) large injury currents were flowing across the ischemic border, which exerted a depolarizing effect on the normal tissue adjacent to the border zone, just before earliest ectopic activity was recorded in that area.

2.1. *Injury currents*

As a consequence of the potential differences between the intercellular compartments of ischemic and normal cells, local current circuits are set up across the ischemic border, provided ischemic and nonischemic cells are well coupled. These so called injury currents change direction and have different magnitudes in the various phases of the cardiac cycle. In diastole, for example, due to the partial depolarization of ischemic cells, the intracellular compartments within the ischemic zone are positive with respect to the intracellular space in the nonischemic part of the heart. Therefore, an intracellular current will flow from ischemic towards normal cells; this current crosses the cell membranes and flows through the extracellular space in the opposite direction, giving rise to a negative extracellular potential in the ischemic area (TQ segment depression) and a positive potential in the normal part of

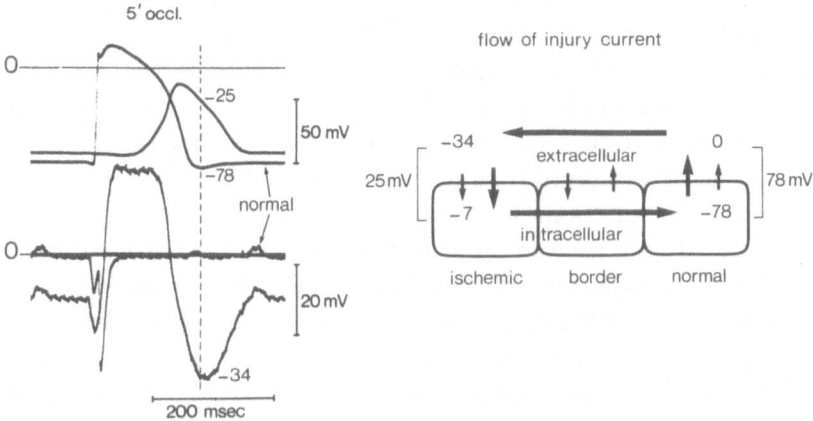

Figure 12. Transmembrane potentials and extracellular complexes from the control situation, and after 5 min of coronary artery occlusion in an isolated dog heart, are superimposed. Schematic diagram shows flow of intra- and extracellular currents at the moment indicated by the vertical dotted line. This injury current, which flows when ischemic cells display delayed repolarization and normal cells have already repolarized, exerts a depolarizing effect on normal cells close to the border. (Reproduced with permission from M.J. Janse et al. In: Management of Ventricular Tachycardia; Role of Mexiletine. Edit. E. Sandoe, D.G. Julian, J.W. Bellpp. 183–196. Amsterdam: Excerpta Medica, 1978.)

the heart (TQ segment elevation). In systole, because of the smaller amplitude of the action potentials of ischemic cells, the intracellular potential difference between normal and ischemic cells has an opposite sign: intracellular current flows from normal towards ischemic cells, and extracellular current flows from the ischemic area towards the normal part of the heart, resulting in ST segment elevation in the ischemic area and ST segment depression in the nonischemic part.

The largest currents flow across the ischemic border in the situation which is depicted in Figure 12. In the left-hand part of the Figure, transmembrane potentials (upper row) of an ischemic cell and a normal cell are superimposed, together with the corresponding local DC-extracellular electrograms (lower row). As common time reference, the P wave was taken. Due to the delayed activation of the ischemic cell, its depolarization occurs at the moment when the normal cell has already repolarized, and has recovered its excitability. At that moment a large current, indicated by the dotted line, flows across the border, as schematically indicated by the right part of the Figure. This current will tend to depolarize the normal cells, and as these have regained their excitability, the current might re-excite the normal cells so as to give rise to an extrasystole. It can be seen that in this situation, i.e. a state of delayed activation of ischemic cells leading to delayed repolarization, a deep negative deflection is recorded in the extracellular space of the ischemic zone; at that moment, current sources are present in the extracellular space on the normal part of the border, but current sinks in the extracellular space on the ischemic side of the border. By measuring DC potentials at many extracellular sites from regularly spaced electrodes, we could construct isopotential maps at any desired moment of the cardiac cycle. From such maps, the distribution of current sinks (transmembrane current flowing into cells) and current sources (transmembrane current flowing out of cells) could be calculated [4]. It turned out that in a situation as outlined above, when deep negative 'T waves' were present in the ischemic area just before ectopic activity emerged from the non-ischemic side of the border, current sources on the normal side of the border were in the order of 2 $\mu A/mm^3$. This figure must be compared with the current sources which are associated with the propagation of activity in normal myocardium. When a broad wavefront travels through normal tissue, local current circuits are set up: in the extracellular space of the tissue about to be excited by the propagating wavefront, current sources in the order of 5 $\mu A/mm^3$ were found. In other words, the injury current flowing across the ischemic border, just before the emergence of a spontaneous premature beat, is about half as strong as the electrotonic currents associated with propagation of a broad wavefront, having a large safety margin, through normal myocardium.

The hypothesis that injury currents may play a role in the genesis of ventricular arrhythmias in acute ischemia is not new [2, 31]. The exact mechanism by which injury currents might induce ventricular premature beats is not established. The various possibilities are: 1) re-excitation during the repolarization phase of normal myocardial or Purkinje cells, which are in electrotonic contact with ischemic cells displaying delayed repolarization; 2) the induction of early or delayed after-depolarizations in either myocardial or Purkinje cells, which could result in abnormal automatic activity [32, 33]. Finally, the possibility cannot be excluded that micro re-entry [34] or reflection [35] within small areas (i.e. several mm) in the ischemic border zone are responsible for the genesis of ventricular premature beats.

3. ANTIARRHYTHMIC ACTION OF DRUGS

Since the nature of the 'focal' mechanism responsible for the occurrence of premature beats is not yet known, speculations about antiarrhythmic actions to suppress this mechanism will not be made here, and only those actions will be considered which could prevent re-entry.

One of the major requirements for re-entry is the presence of a zone, or zones, of unidirectional block. In acutely ischemic myocardium not all cells will be affected to the same degree. As already described, differences of only a few mV in resting membrane potential between adjacent cell groups will lead to marked disparities in refractory periods. Premature beats, or normally propagated beats when heart rate is increased, can therefore be expected to be blocked in certain areas and to be conducted slowly in others, thus setting the stage for re-entry.

In principle, re-entry can be abolished in two ways: either by further depressing excitability, and so converting areas of unidirectional block into areas of bidirectional block, or by improving the electrical activity and changing the zone of unidirectional block into tissue which will conduct the impulse.

We have already seen that lidocaine has an extra depressant effect on the upstroke characteristics of the action potentials of ischemic cells. Lidocaine increases the area within the ischemic myocardium which is inexcitable, even during moderately slow heart rates, and accelerates the transition from depressed conduction to failure of activation. In other words, lidocaine converted areas of unidirectional block into zones of total block. At the same time, conduction delay in those ischemic areas where conduction persisted was greater in the presence of lidocaine than in the absence of it [16]. Thus, the slowing of conduction together with the extension of the area of total block create the conditions for circus movement with a large diameter, but abolish conditions for micro re-entry and fragmentation of wavefronts into multiple wavelets travelling through multiple islands of partial conduction block.

In our experiments [16], a low concentration of lidocaine (1 μg/ml) had no effect on the incidence of arrhythmias during coronary occlusion. When a high dosage (5 μg/ml) was administered prior to an occlusion, the incidence of ventricular premature beats and runs of ventricular tachycardia was no different from that during control occlusions. However, the incidence of ventricular fibrillation was significantly reduced: it occurred only once in a heart that was paced at a rapid rate, out of a series of 13 hearts (in control occlusions in the same hearts, fibrillation occurred 8 times). The arrhythmogenic effect of fast heart rates in acute ischemia in the experimental animal has been emphasized by Scherlag et al. [36]. An increase in heart rate may unmask slight differences in recovery properties in adjacent cell groups so that propagation fails in those cells with a more advanced degree of post-repolarization refractoriness, and slow conduction is still possible in slightly less depressed cells. In this way the stage may be set for multiple wavelet re-entry. It is possible that in the presence of lidocaine, at a time when excitability is reduced but not yet abolished in the greater part of the ischemic zone, the arrhythmogenic effect of the fast heart rate overrules the antiarrhythmic effect of lidocaine. In this respect it is noteworthy that in the very early phase of myocardial infarction, lidocaine was found to be less effective in the presence of sinus tachycardia [37].

The pattern of activation during two arrhythmias occurring in the same heart during two successive occlusions, is shown in Figure 13. In the control occlusion (upper row) in the absence of the drug, ventricular fibrillation occurred spontaneously after several minutes. The position of the multiple electrode is shown in the right panel, every dot indicating an individual electrode terminal. Also shown are isopotential lines, based on DC potential measurements during the TQ segment of a beat propagated from the atrium. The zero potential line marks the position of the electrophysiological border zone. During the first ectopic beat (time zero is the P wave of the last propagated beat) earliest activity was found in the normal myocardium close to the apex. (A second wavefront invaded the ischemic area from the right ventricle, but since only a few electrode terminals were located there it could not be ascertained whether this wavefront also originated outside the ischemic area.) In the next beats, similar activation patterns were found (not shown), but

62

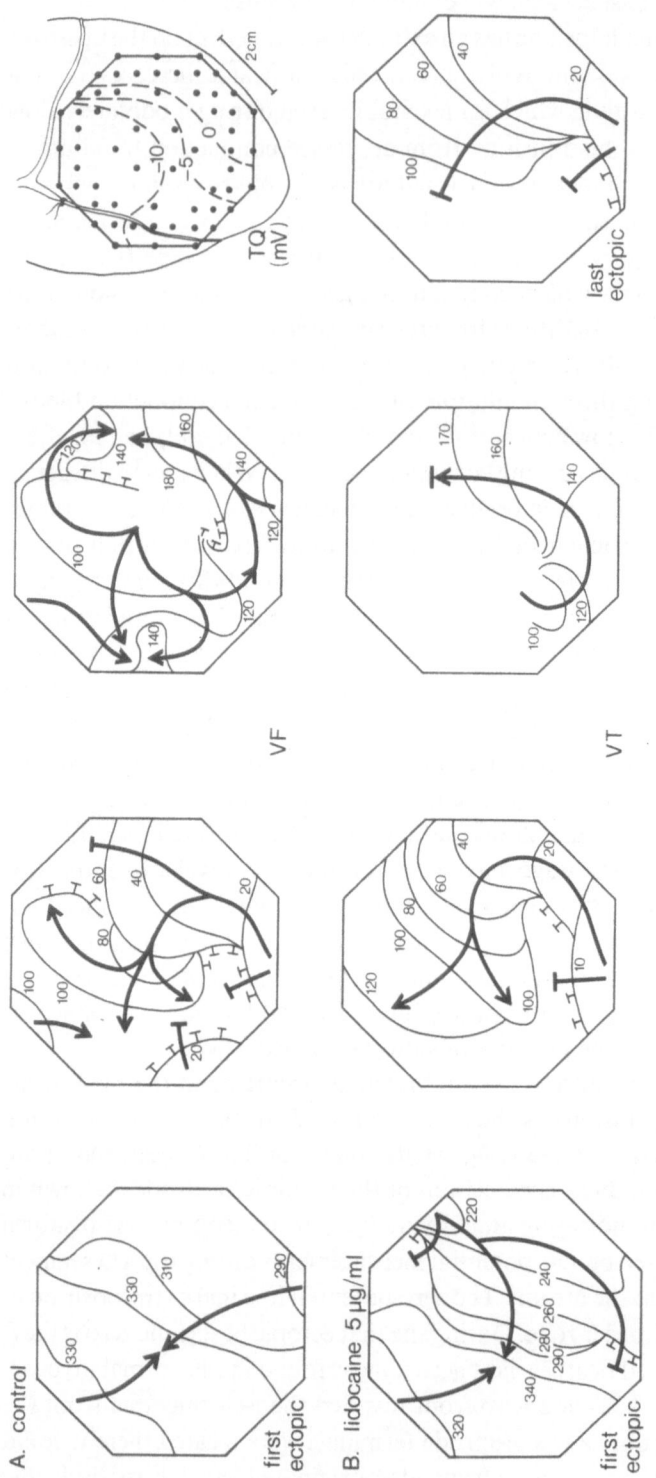

Figure 13. Effects of lidocaine on patterns of activation during spontaneous ventricular arrhythmias in the first minutes after coronary occlusion. In the control occlusion, a spontaneous ventricular premature beat (left panel) triggered a tachycardia which eventually changed into ventricular fibrillation (middle panels). In the upper right panel, the position of the multiple electrode on the heart is indicated, as are isopotential lines during the TQ segment of a normally propagated beat. In the presence of lidocaine (lower row), premature beats and tachycardias still occurred and circus movement re-entry was occasionally observed, but no fragmentation into multiple wavelets re-entry occurred. (Reproduced with permission of [16].)

gradually, islands of conduction block appeared, and finally the activation pattern shown in the middle two panels emerged. Multiple activation waves were present, one of which described a complete circus movement with a diameter of less than 1 cm. Other wavefronts described incomplete circus movements, and both collision and fusion of wavefronts occurred. The heart was defibrillated, and the occlusion released. Lidocaine (5 μg/ml) was added to the perfusion fluid, and 15 min later, another occlusion was performed. After a few minutes, a ventricular premature beat (first ectopic, shown in the lower left panel) initiated a long run of ventricular tachycardia (54 ectopic impulses) which terminated spontaneously. In the initial beats, earliest activity was again found on the non-ischemic side of the border, and this remained so in later beats. However, on occasion, circus movements of fairly large diameters were found to occur. In the middle two panels, the activation sequences during beats 35 and 36 are shown (time zero was arbitrarily chosen). A wavefront originating from the apical area was blocked in its way to the center of the ischemic zone, and conducted in the border zone and the non-ischemic tissue in a counter clockwise fashion. After one and a half revolutions, the wavefront was blocked. This activation pattern showed some similarity with the patterns shown in the upper two middle panels, but no multiple wavelets were present. In the very last (54th) beat of the tachycardia, early activity again emerged from the non-ischemic myocardium; an attempted circus movement was described which was blocked after only one half of a revolution. Thereafter, sinus rhythm was restored.

During tachycardias recorded in the absence of the drug, in different experiments, 21 instances of successful circus movement re-entry were mapped in 18 ectopic beats. All these tachycardias degenerated into ventricular fibrillation. In contrast, during ventricular tachycardia in the same hearts in the presence of lidocaine (5 μg/ml), only 7 instances of successful circus movement re-entry were found in 62 ectopic beats. All of these tachycardias terminated spontaneously.

In epicardial preparations excised from infarcted hearts 1–3 days after coronary occlusion [17], lidocaine had similar effects as in our studies on acute ischemic myocardium. These authors also concluded that 'lidocaine owes its antiarrhythmic potency to the abolition of markedly depressed responses and extinguishment of very slow conduction.'

On the other hand, if electrical activity in ischemic tissue would improve (i.e. if action potentials would have larger amplitudes and faster upstrokes, and the cells would not exhibit post-repolarization refractoriness) multiplewavelet re-entry leading to ventricular fibrillation would also vanish. In agreement with the findings of Elharrar et al. [38] and Fondacaro et al. [39], we found that verapamil improved conduction in the ischemic myocardium in the early phase of ischemia. Our experiments, because of the limited number of hearts studied, do not allow for any conclusion to be drawn about the effect of verapamil on the incidence of arrhythmias, but in the two studies mentioned above, a reduction in the incidence of ventricular arrhythmias was observed. Whether an improvement in conduction in the ischemic myocardium always has an antiarrhythmic effect is to be doubted.

Reperfusion, which quickly restores conduction in previously unresponsive myocardium, is one of the most effective ways to induce ventricular fibrillation.

Preliminary experiments in our laboratory have indicated that left stellate ganglion stimulation during coronary occlusion in dog hearts in situ markedly improves conduction in ischemic myocardium, and transforms areas of block into areas of conduction. Yet, as in previous studies [40, 41], left stellate ganglion stimulation in the very early phase of ischemia was in our experiments highly arrhythmogenic. It is of course possible that sympathetic stimulation would primarily affect the 'focal' mechanism responsible for the genesis of (multiple) premature beats, whether this would be abnormal automaticity or triggered automaticity due to enhancement of either early or late after-depolarizations [32, 42], and have little effect on the re-entrant component of the ventricular arrhythmias.

It might be fruitful to direct future research towards unravelling the nature of the 'focal' mechanism, and to find ways of influencing it by pharmacological means. At present, the most effective way to suppress the re-entrant component would be to depress maximally electrical activity within the ischemic myocardium so that the occurrence of multiple wavelet re-entry is prevented.

ACKNOWLEDGEMENTS

This study was supported by a grant from the Wynand Pon Foundation in Amsterdam.

REFERENCES

1. Harris AS, Rojas AG: The initiation of ventricular fibrillation due to coronary occlusion. Exp Med Surg 1:105–122, 1943.
2. Harris AS: Delayed development of ventricular ectopic rhythms following experimental coronary occlusion. Circulation 1:1318–1328, 1950.
3. Stephenson SE, Cole RK, Parrish TF, Bauer FM, Johnson IT, Kochitzky M, Anderson JS, Hibbitt LL, McCarty IE, Young ER, Wilson JR, Meiers NH, Neador CK, Ball OT, Neneely GR: Ventricular fibrillation during and after coronary artery occlusion. Incidence and protection afforded by drugs. Am J Cardiol 5:77–87, 1960.
4. Janse MJ, van Capelle FJL, Morsink H, Kléber AG, Wilms-Schopman F, Cardinal R, Naumann d'Alnoncourt C, Durrer D: Flow of 'injury' current and patterns of excitation during early ventricular arrhythmias in acute regional myocardial ischemia in isolated porcine and canine hearts. Evidence for two arrhythmogenic mechanisms. Circ Res 47:151–165, 1980.
5. Bigger JT, Dresdale RJ, Heissenbuttel RH, Weld FM, Wit AL: Ventricular arrhythmias in ischemic heart disease: mechanism, prevalence, significance and management. Progr Cardiovasc Dis 19:255–300, 1977.
6. Pantridge JF, Webb SW, Adgey AAJ: Arrhythmias in the first hours of acute myocardial infarction. Progr Cardiovasc Dis 23:265–277, 1981.
7. Scherlag BJ, El-Sherif N, Hope RR, Lazzara R: Characterization and localization of ventricular arrhythmias resulting from myocardial ischemia and infarction. Circ Res 35:372–383, 1974.

65

8. Kaplinsky E, Ogawa S, Balke CW, Dreifus LS: Two periods of early ventricular arrhythmias in the canine acute myocardial infarction model. Circulation 60:397–403, 1979.
9. Harris AS, Bisteni A, Russell RA, Brightam JC, Firestone JE: Excitable factors in ventricular tachycardia resulting from myocardial ischemia: potassium a major excitant. Science 199:200–203, 1954.
10. Hill JL, Gettes LS: Effect of acute coronary artery occlusion on local myocardial extracellular K$^+$ activity in swine. Circulation 61:768–778, 1980.
11. Hirche HJ, Franz C, Bös L, Bissig R, Lang R, Schramm M: Myocardial extracellular K$^+$ and H$^+$ increase and noradrenaline release as possible cause of early arrhythmias following acute coronary artery occlusion in pigs. J Moll Cell Cardiol 12:579–593, 1980.
12. Carmeliet E: Cardiac transmembrane potentials and metabolism. Circ Res 42:577–587, 1978.
13. Weidmann S: The effect of the cardiac membrane potential on the rapid availability of the sodium carrying system. J Physiol (Lond) 127:213–224, 1955.
14. Moréna H, Janse MJ, Fiolet JWT, Krieger WJG, Crijns H, Durrer D:Comparison of the effects of regional ischemia, hypoxia, hyperkalemia and acidosis on intracellular and extracellular potentials and metabolism in the isolated porcine heart. Circ Res 46:634–646, 1980.
15. Brennan JF, Cranefield PF, Wit AL: Effects of lidocaine on slow response and depressed fast response action potentials of canine cardiac Purkinje fibers. J Pharmacol Exp Ther 204:312–324, 1978.
16. Cardinal R, Janse MJ, Eeden J van, Werner G, Naumann d'Alnoncourt C, Durrer D: The effects of lidocaine on intracellular and extracellular potentials, activation and ventricular arrhythmias during acute regional ischemia in the intact isolated porcine heart. Circ Res 49:792–806, 1981.
17. Lazzara R, Hope RR, El-Sherif N, Scherlag BJ: Effects of lidocaine on hypoxic and ischemic cardiac cells. Am J Cardiol 41:872–879, 1978.
18. Kléber AG, Janse MJ, van Capelle FLJ, Durrer D: Mechanism and time course of S-T and T-Q segment changes during acute regional myocardial ischemia in the pig heart determined by extracellular and intracellular recordings. Circ Res 42:603–613, 1978.
19. Downar E, Janse MJ, Durrer D: The effect of acute coronary artery occlusion on subepicardial transmembrane potentials in the intact porcine heart. Circulation 56:217–224, 1977.
20. Cinca J, Janse MJ, Moréna H, Candell J, Valle V, Durrer D: Mechanism and time course of the early electrical changes during acute coronary artery occlusion. An attempt to correlate the early ECG changes in man to the cellular electrophysiology in the pig. Chest 77:499–505, 1980.
21. Mascher D: Electrical and mechanical responses from ventricular muscle fibers after inactivation of the sodium carrying system. Pfluegers Arch 317:359–372, 1970.
22. Schneider JA, Sperelakis N: The demonstration of energy dependence of the isoproterenol-induced transcellular Ca^{2+} current in isolated perfused guinea pig hearts. An explanation for mechanical failure of ischemic myocardium. J Surg Res 16:389–403, 1974.
23. Bassingthwaighte JB, Fry CH, McGuigan JAS: Relationship between internal calcium and outward current in mammalian ventricular muscle; a mechanism for the control of the action potential duration? J Physiol (Lond) 262:15–27, 1976.
24. Brooks C McC, Gilbert JL, Greenspan ME, Lange G, Mazzella HM: Excitability and electrical response of ischemic heart muscle. Am J Physiol 198:1143–1147, 1960.
25. Lazzara R, El-Sherif N, Hope RR, Scherlag BJ: Ventricular arrhythmias and electrophysiological consequences of myocardial ischemia and infarction. Circ Res 42:740–749, 1978.
26. Schütz E: Elektrophysiologie des Herzens bei einphasische Ableitung. Ergebn Physiol 38:493–620, 1936.
27. Hoffman BF, Cranefield PF: The Electrophysiology of the Heart. New York: McGraw Hill, 1960.
28. Gettes LS, Reuter H: Slow recovery from inactivation of inward currents in mammalian myocardial fibers. J Physiol (Lond) 240:703–724, 1974.
29. van Capelle FJL, Morsink H, Janse MJ, Durrer D: Computerized DC epicardial mapping during experimental coronary occlusion. Comput Cardiol IEEE Sept:99–102, 1979.

66

30. Moe GK: On the multiple wavelet hypothesis of atrial fibrillation. Arch Int Pharmacodyn Ther 140:183–188, 1962.
31. Hoffman BF: The genesis of cardiac arrhythmias. Progr Cardiovasc Dis 8:319–329, 1966.
32. Cranefield PF: The Conduction of the Cardiac Impulse. Mount Kisco, New York: Futura Publishing Co, 1975.
33. Katzung BG, Hondghem LM, Grant AO: Cardiac ventricular automaticity induced by current of injury. Pfluegers Arch 360:193–197, 1975.
34. Wit AL, Cranefield PF, Hoffman BF: Slow conduction and re-entry in the ventricular conducting system. II. Single and sustained circus movements in networks of canine and bovine Purkinje fibers. Circ Res 30:11–22, 1972.
35. Antzelevitch C, Jalife J, Moe GK: Characteristics of reflection as a mechanism of re-entrant arrhythmias and its relationship to parasystole. Circulation 61:182–191, 1980.
36. Scherlag BJ, Helfant RH, Haft JT, Damato AN: Electrophysiology underlying ventricular arrhythmias due to coronary ligation. Am J Physiol 219:1665–1672, 1970.
37. Adgey AAJ, Webb SW: The treatment of ventricular arrhythmias in acute myocardial infarction. Br J Hosp Med 21:356–379, 1979.
38. Elharrar V, Gaum WE, Zipes DP: Effect of drugs on conduction delay and incidence of ventricular arrhythmias induced by acute coronary occlusion in dogs. Am J Cardiol 39:544–549, 1977.
39. Fondacaro JD, Han J, Yoon MS: Effects of verapamil on ventricular rhythm during acute coronary occlusion. Am Heart J 96:81–86, 1978.
40. Harris AS, Otero H, Bocage AJ: The induction of arrhythmias by sympathetic activity before and after occlusion of a coronary artery in the canine heart. J Electrocardiol 4:34–43, 1971.
41. Rosenfeld J, Rosen MR, Hoffman BF: Pharmacologic and behavioral effects on arrhythmias which immediately follow coronary occlusion: a canine model of sudden death. Am J Cardiol 41:1075–1082, 1978.
42. Hoffman BF: Role of the sympathetic nervous system in arrhythmias occurring after coronary artery occlusion and myocardial infarction. In: Neural Mechanisms in Cardiac Arrhythmias. (PJ Schwartz, AM Brown, A Malliani, A. Zanchetti eds.) pp. 155–165. New York: Raven Press, 1978.

4. INITIATION OF VENTRICULAR FIBRILLATION OUTSIDE HOSPITAL

A.A. JENNIFER ADGEY

The mechanism of arrhythmias following acute infarction, whether enhanced automaticity or re-entry or both, appears to vary depending on the time after coronary occlusion. Early after myocardial infarction, ventricular fibrillation may result from re-entrant excitation. During the later stages of infarction enhanced automaticity may precipitate ventricular fibrillation. Janse et al. have suggested that, within the first 15 minutes following experimental coronary occlusion, the premature beat is initiated by injury currents [1]. By its prematurity this beat increases the differences in conduction velocity and refractory periods of ischemic and non-ischemic tissue in the border zone and creates the conditions where micro re-entry can exist. It is probable that minute differences in the way the premature beat is conducted may decide whether or not re-entry succeeds.

Although sudden cardiac death claims approximately 1200 lives daily in the USA, and although it is the leading cause of death among men aged 20–64 years, many aspects of sudden death still remain unsolved. Factors initiating the sudden collapse or ventricular fibrillation are largely unknown since ventricular fibrillation rarely develops in the community in the presence of continuous electrocardiographic monitoring. Many sudden deaths are instantaneous. Thus, the majority of patients are in ventricular fibrillation when first seen. Pantridge et al. found that among patients with primary ventricular fibrillation during the first hour of myocardial infarction, 82% were in ventricular fibrillation before the mobile team arrived [2]. Factors which may initiate ventricular fibrillation have been assessed in patients who developed it outside hospital after the arrival of the Belfast Mobile Coronary Care Unit. Excluded from the study were patients who were either in ventricular fibrillation or sustained ventricular tachycardia when first seen.

Forty-eight consecutive patients who developed ventricular fibrillation outside hospital were studied. Forty were male, aged 37–79 years (mean age 56 years), and 8 were female aged 40–76 (mean age 59 years). The site of infarction was anterior in 29 (63%), inferior in 15 (33%); in one anterior and inferior and subendocardial in one. One patient had myocardial ischemia and aortic stenosis was present in the remaining patient. Thirteen patients had had one or more previous myocardial infarctions. Thirty-nine patients had primary ventricular fibrillation. The median time from onset of symptoms of myocardial infarction to arrival of the mobile coronary care unit was 68 min. Twenty-two patients were seen within one hour. The median time from onset of symptoms to development of ventricular fibrillation was

Adgey, AAJ (ed): Acute phase of ischemic heart disease and myocardial infarction.
© *1982, Martinus Nijhoff, The Hague, Boston, London. ISBN-13: 978-94-009-7581-1*

Table 1. Initial and pre-ventricular fibrillation heart rates in the 48 patients

Initial	47–175/min (mean 84 ± 4.14 SEM)
Pre-VF	52–214/min (mean 98 ± 4.99 SEM)
Paired t test P < 0.001	

105 min. Ten patients developed ventricular fibrillation within one hour. Thirty-five patients (73%) survived to leave hospital.

1. HEART RHYTHM AND RATE

On arrival, 25 patients were in sinus rhythm, 10 had sinus tachycardia, and 10 had sinus bradycardia; atrial fibrillation was present in 2 patients, and second degree atrio-ventricular block in 1 patient. The blood pressure was recorded in 42 patients. The range of systolic pressures was 60–195 mm Hg (mean 124 mm Hg). In 6 patients, it was not possible to take a blood pressure recording since the speed of development of ventricular fibrillation precluded the estimation of the blood pressure. The electrocardiographic monitoring time prior to the development of ventricular fibrillation varied from 1 to 80 min (mean 25 min). The rhythm and blood pressure recorded immediately preceding ventricular fibrillation did not differ significantly from that recorded initially.

From the electrocardiographic tape recordings, three specific heart rates were obtained: 1) the heart rate when the patient was first seen and connected to the tape recorder (initial); 2) the heart rate immediately preceding ventricular fibrillation (pre-ventricular fibrillation); 3) the heart rate immediately prior to movement in patients who developed ventricular fibrillation on movement, or in the ambulance during the journey to hospital (pre-movement). The range of the initial heart rates, and those pre-ventricular fibrillation are recorded in Table 1. There was a significant increase in the heart rates immediately prior to ventricular fibrillation (paired t test of the differences between the initial and pre-ventricular fibrillation heart rates, P < 0.001). On excluding those patients who had received atropine or a beta-blocking agent, the P value was still significant (P < 0.01). Figure 1 shows the distribution of the initial and pre-ventricular fibrillation heart rates. An increase in heart rate is shown for the majority of patients. In 12 of the 48 patients, ventricular fibrillation occurred during movement of the patient from the position when first seen (Table 2). There was a significant increase between the initial and pre-movement heart rates and between the initial and pre-ventricular fibrillation heart rates.

1.1. Autonomic disturbance

Alteration in the para-sympathetic and sympathetic nervous systems is important in

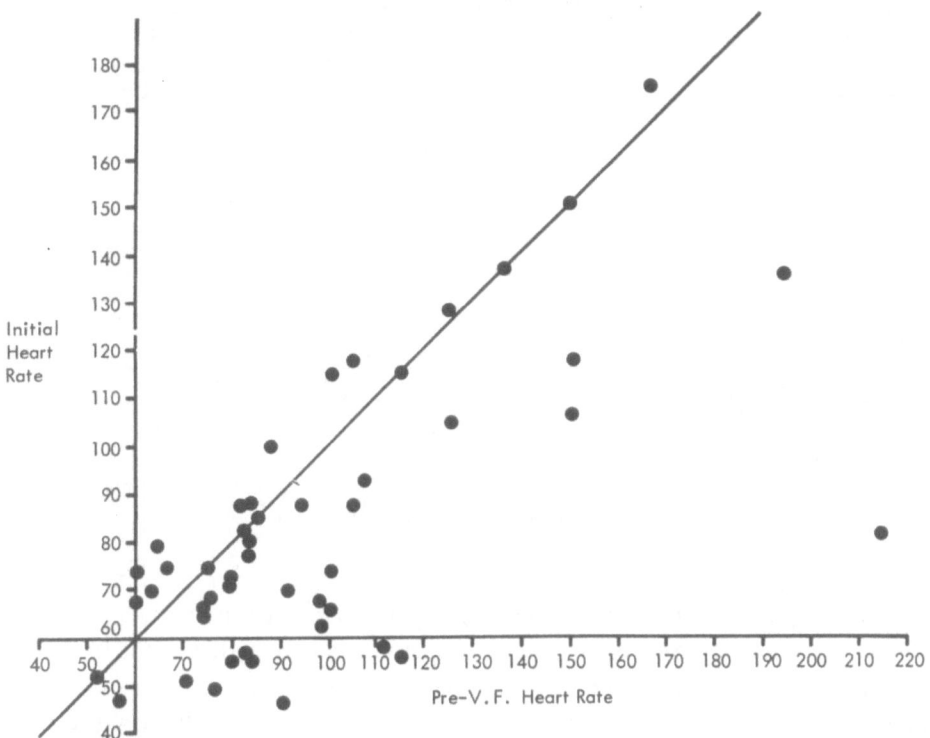

Figure 1. Initial and pre-ventricular fibrillation heart rates in the 48 patients. The line drawn represents a heart rate of no change.

the genesis of arrhythmias within the early hours of the acute coronary event. Clinical and experimental studies have shown that ventricular fibrillation may be associated with extremes of heart rate – bradycardia and tachycardia [2–4]. Parasympathetic overactivity, most frequently associated with a diaphragmatic infarction, is present in 48% of patients seen within 30 min of the onset of symptoms, and sympathetic overactivity, most frequently associated with anterior infarction, is present in 35% of patients seen within a similar time period [2]. During the movement of patients with acute myocardial infarction and despite analgesia, a heart rate of $\geqslant 100$/min has been recorded in 45% [5].

Table 2. Initial, pre-movement and pre-ventricular fibrillation heart rates in 12 patients where ventricular fibrillation occurred during movement

A. Initial heart rate	48–136/min (mean 85 ± 8.96 SEM)
B. Pre-movement heart rate	48–152/min (mean 95.5 ± 9.96 SEM)
C. Pre-VF heart rate	56–194/min (mean 104 ± 11.06 SEM)
Paired t test between A. and B.	0.05 > P > 0.025
Paired t test between A. and C.	0.02 > P > 0.01

70

Table 3. Ectopic activity prior to initiation of ventricular fibrillation

	No. of patients	Incidence %
Late cycle ventricular ectopics	38	79
R on T ventricular ectopics	27	56
Consecutive ventricular ectopics	14	29
Multifocal ventricular ectopics	3	6
Bigeminal ventricular ectopics	3	6
VT (self-terminating)	3	6
Atrial ectopics	3	6
No ectopic activity	6	12

Consecutive ventricular ectopics – two successive ventricular ectopics occurring in pairs.
Bigeminal ventricular ectopics – a ventricular ectopic alternating with a normally conducted beat for at least two normally conducted beats.
VT (self-terminating) ventricular tachycardia – three or more successive ventricular ectopics at a ventricular rate of > 120/min and self-terminating. Reproduced with permission [26].

Increased plasma catecholamine levels have been reported in animals following left anterior descending coronary artery occlusion and in man during the first hour of acute myocardial infarction [6, 7]. Sympathetic overactivity in association with acute myocardial infarction may cause a fall in the ventricular fibrillation threshold [8], predispose to ventricular dysrhythmias [2] and since heart rate is a major determinant of myocardial oxygen demand, an increase in the extent of myocardial ischemic injury [9]. When beta-blockers are administered in the experimental situation, the incidence of ventricular fibrillation has been reduced [10, 11]. In this study, the heart rhythm immediately preceding ventricular fibrillation did not differ significantly from that reported when the patient was seen initially, but there was a significant increase in the heart rate from the time the patient was first seen until that recorded immediately prior to ventricular fibrillation. This was so even after excluding patients who had received prior treatment with atropine or beta-blocking agents. When ventricular fibrillation occurred during the movement of a patient to hospital there was also a significant increase in heart rate from that recorded initially.

2. WARNING ARRHYTHMIAS

The significance of 'warning' or premonitory arrhythmias which antecede the development of ventricular fibrillation, still gives rise to major debate. The generally accepted criteria for 'warning arrhythmias' are ventricular ectopics falling into one of the following four categories: 1) R on T, 2) > 5/minute, 3) multi-focal, 4) coupled or in salvos. In experimental and clinical studies, R on T ectopics have been reported with varying frequency. A study in baboons showed that 69% who developed

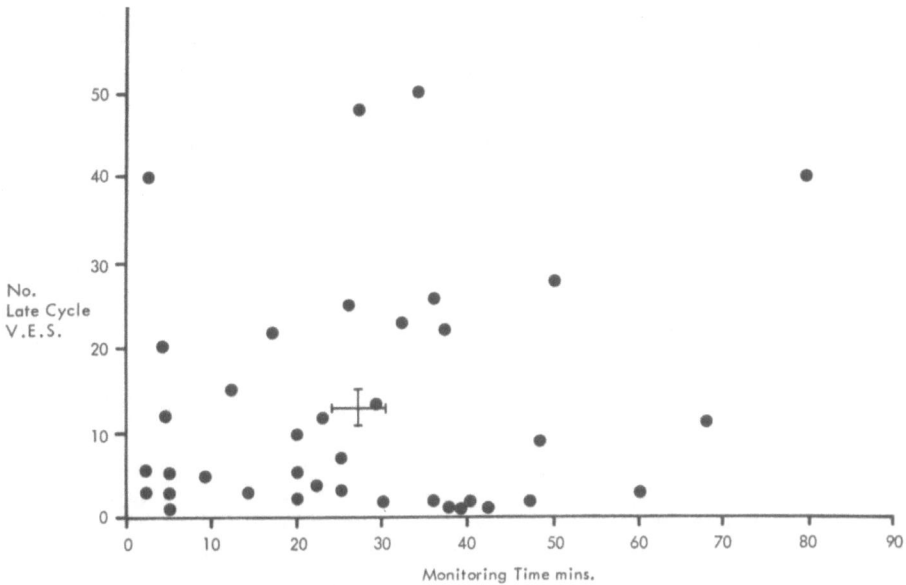

Figure 2. Frequency distribution of late cycle ventricular ectopics (38 patients) in relation to monitoring time (mean 13 late cycle ventricular ectopics for average monitoring time of 27 min.)

ventricular fibrillation within the first hour of acute myocardial infarction had R on T ectopics [12]. Lie et al. found that of patients admitted within 6 h of the onset of infarction, only 10% of those who developed primary ventricular fibrillation had R on T ectopics as 'warning arrhythmias' [13]. El-Sherif et al. showed that of those with primary ventricular fibrillation, occurring in the majority within 24 h of the onset of infarction, only 25% had antecedent R on T ectopics [14]. It is of interest that in these two studies [13, 14] as many patients had R on T ectopics with subsequent development of ventricular fibrillation as those who did not.

It may well be that the pattern or timing of ventricular ectopics as 'warning arrhythmias' is not necessarily crucial to the development of ventricular fibrillation but the capacity of the infarcted ventricle to sustain repetitive beating. In this study, ectopic activity during the premonitory phase but excluding that initiating ventricular fibrillation was recorded (Table 3). The prematurity index of ventricular premature beats was assessed by dividing the coupling interval of the ventricular premature beat (RR') by the QT interval of the preceding normally conducted beat. A ventricular ectopic beat with a prematurity index of < 1 was considered to represent the R on T phenomenon, while a premature beat with an index of $\geqslant 1$ was termed long-coupling or late cycle. Late cycle ventricular ectopics were the most frequent, occurring in 38 (79%) patients. The frequency distribution of late cycle ventricular ectopics in relation to the monitoring time is shown in Figure 2. The average number of late cycle ventricular ectopics recorded was 13 for a mean monitoring time of 27 min. However, many patients with ischemic heart disease

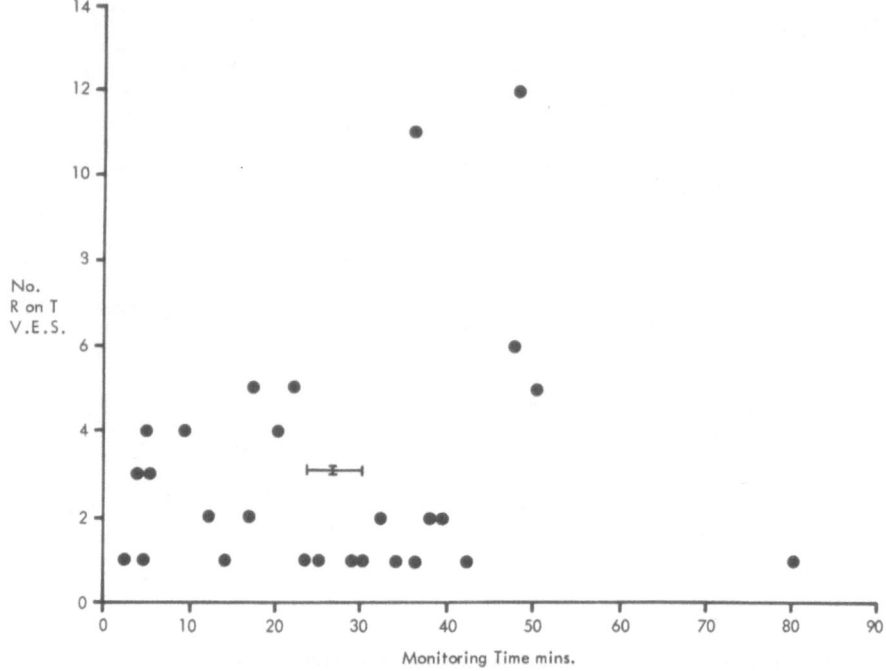

Figure 3. Frequency distribution of R on T ectopics (27 patients) in relation to monitoring time (mean 3 R on T ectopics for average monitoring time of 27 min).

uncomplicated by ventricular fibrillation have late cycle ectopics. R on T ventricular ectopics were present in 27 (56%) patients. However, only an average of 3 R on T ectopics were recorded during a mean monitoring time of 27 min (Figure 3). Multi-focal, consecutive or bigeminal ventricular ectopics and atrial ectopics were relatively infrequent. Ventricular ectopics occurring with a frequency of >5/min were rare. In some patients a burst of ventricular ectopics immediately preceded the initiation of ventricular fibrillation (Figure 4). Sustained ventricular tachycardia is rare during the early phase of acute myocardial infarction.In this study, self-terminating ventricular tachycardia (at least three or more successive ventricular ectopics occurring at a ventricular rate of >120/min) prior to the development of ventricular fibrillation, occurred in 6%. In 6 patients no ventricular ectopic activity was recorded. They had a shorter average monitoring time (9 min) than that of the whole group.

The time from the development of 'warning arrhythmias' to ventricular fibrillation was very short in many cases and this precluded the institution of anti-arrhythmic therapy. It therefore calls into question the significance of 'warning arrhythmias' in the administration of anti-arrhythmic therapy.

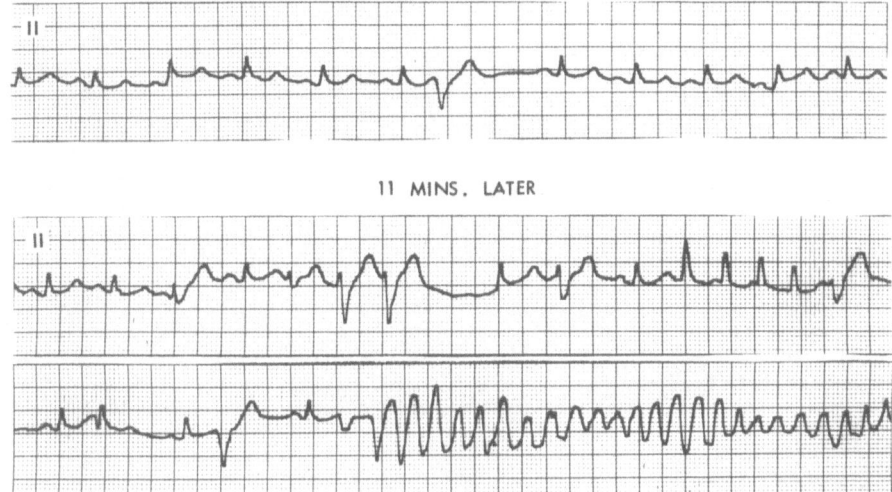

11 MINS. LATER

Figure 4. Top tracing – single R on T ectopic during out of hospital monitoring, heart rate less than 100/min (Lead II EKG). Eleven minutes after top tracing, heart rate increased, burst of late cycle and R on T ectopics ending in ventricular fibrillation (second and third tracings continuous). Reproduced with permission [26].

3. INITIATION OF VENTRICULAR FIBRILLATION

Major controversy still surrounds the initiation of ventricular fibrillation. Wiggers [15], and Wiggers and Wegria [16] first noted that animals were most vulnerable to ventricular fibrillation when very short condenser shocks were delivered during late systole, i.e. within the T wave or 'vulnerable phase.' The clinical significance of the vulnerable phase (R on T) was first emphasised by Smirk and Palmer [17]. The study by Dhurandhar et al. [18] showed that an R on T ectopic was the initiating beat in 80% of those who developed primary ventricular fibrillation. In similar studies by Lie et al. [13] and El-Sherif et al. [14] the initiating beat was an R on T ectopic in 45% and 50% of the cases, respectively. Nevertheless, clinical and experimental work has shown that ventricular fibrillation may be initiated by an R on T or a late cycle ectopic [19, 20]. In this study an R on T ectopic was the most important factor in the initiation of ventricular fibrillation: it was found in 33 of the 48 patients (69%) (Figure 5). A late cycle ventricular ectopic in 3 patients and idioventricular rhythm in a further 3 patients initiated ventricular fibrillation. From ventricular tachycardia, ventricular fibrillation developed in 9 (19%) patients. In a study by Klein et al. [21], of 7 patients with coronary artery disease who suffered sudden death during Holter monitoring, ventricular tachycardia degenerated into ventricular fibrillation in all of them.

74

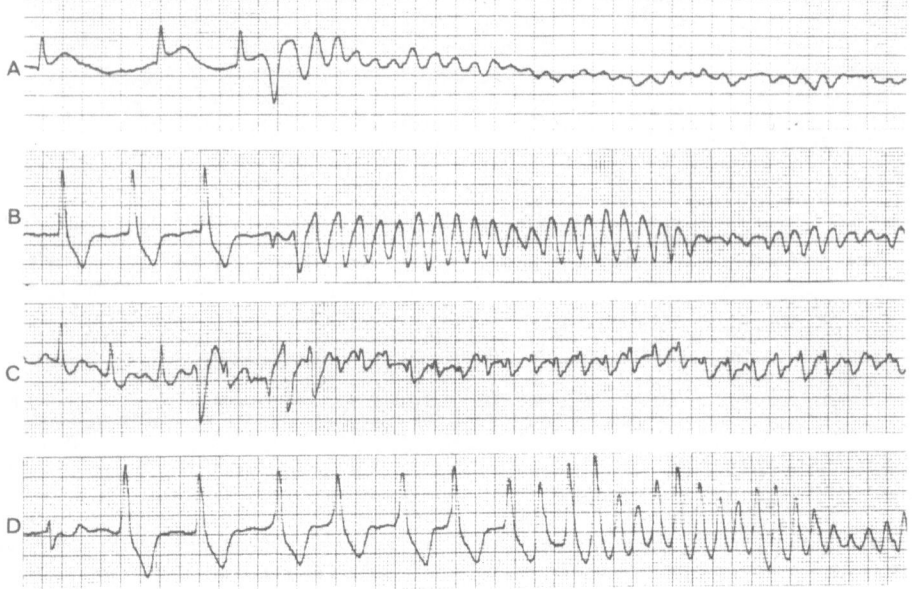

Figure 5. Initiation of ventricular fibrillation.

A. R on T ectopic
B. Late cycle ectopic
C. Ventricular tachycardia/ventricular flutter which degenerated into ventricular fibrillation.
D. Idioventricular rhythm with rapid acceleration into ventricular fibrillation.

4. MYOCARDIAL INFARCTION, MYOCARDIAL ISCHEMIA

Liberthson et al. in a study of long- and short-term survivors from out-of-hospital ventricular fibrillation found that acute myocardial infarction was present in only 39%, and ischemia without infarction in 34% [22]. Baum et al. recorded that in long-term survivors of out-of-hospital ventricular fibrillation, myocardial necrosis based on electrocardiographic or enzyme studies was present in 49.5%, and only 17% had an acute transmural infarction [23]. In 50.5% of their patients there was no evidence of myocardial necrosis. Of the group in ventricular fibrillation when the Seattle Unit arrived, myocardial necrosis was present in 42% and only 10% showed acute transmural infarction. In contrast with those who developed ventricular fibrillation after arrival of the unit, 79% had evidence of myocardial necrosis, and 50% showed acute transmural infarction. In this study where ventricular fibrillation occurred after the arrival of the unit, 96% of short- and long-term survivors had an acute myocardial infarction. The minimum time from onset of symptoms to the development of ventricular fibrillation was 32 min. No patient suffered instantaneous death. It is impossible to say, therefore, that the factors leading to ventricular fibrillation in this group of patients would be identical to those suffering instantaneous death.

4.1. Site of infarction

In this study more patients had an anterior than a diaphragmatic infarction. In the studies of Dhurandhar et al. [18] and El-Sherif et al. [14], anterior infarctions dominated and in the study by Liberthson et al. [22] lesions of the anterior wall dominated, yet in the report of Lie et al. [24] there was a predominance of inferior infarctions. In an earlier study from Belfast, of ventricular fibrillation outside hospital, there was an equal incidence of anterior and inferior infarctions [25].

REFERENCES

1. Janse MJ, Morsink H, Van Capelle FJL, Kleber AG, Wilms-Schopman F, Durrer D: Ventricular arrhythmias in the first 15 minutes of acute regional myocardial ischemia in the isolated pig heart: Possible role of injury currents. In: Sudden Death (Kulbertus HE, Wellens HJJ, eds). Developments in Cardiovascular Medicine. Vol. 4, pp. 89–103. Martinus Nijhoff, The Hague, 1980.
2. Pantridge JF, Webb SW, Adgey AAJ, Geddes JS: The first hour after the onset of acute myocardial infarction. In: Progress in Cardiology. Yu PN, Goodwin JF, eds). Vol. III, pp. 173–188. Lea and Febiger, Philadelphia, 1974.
3. Chadda KD, Banka VS, Helfant RH: Rate dependent ventricular ectopia following acute coronary occlusion. The concept of an optimal antiarrhythmic heart rate. Circulation 49: 645–658, 1974.
4. Scherlag BJ, Helfant RH, Haft JI, Damato AN: Electrophysiology underlying ventricular arrhythmias due to coronary ligation. Am J Physiol 219:1665–71, 1970.
5. Mulholland HC, Pantridge JF: Heart-rate changes during movement of patients with acute myocardial infarction. Lancet 1: 1244–1247, 1974.
6. Staszewska-Barczak J: The reflex stimulation of catecholamine secretion during the acute stage of myocardial infarction in the dog. Clin Sci 41:419–439, 1971.
7. Strange RC, Vetter N, Rowe MJ, Oliver MF: Plasma cyclic AMP and total catecholamines during acute myocardial infarction in man. Eur J Clin Invest 4:115–119, 1974.
8. Kliks BR, Burgess MJ, Abildskov JA: Influence of sympathetic tone on ventricular fibrillation threshold during experimental coronary occlusion. Am J Cardiol 36:45–49, 1975.
9. Redwood DR, Smith ER, Epstein SE: Coronary artery occlusion in the conscious dog: effects of alterations in heart rate and arterial pressure on the degree of myocardial ischaemia. Circulation 46:323–332, 1972.
10. Khan MI, Hamilton JT, Manning GW: Protective effect of beta adrenoceptor blockade in experimental coronary occlusion in conscious dogs. Am J Cardiol 30:832–837, 1972.
11. Khan MI, Hamilton JT, Manning GW: Early arrhythmias following experimental coronary occlusion in conscious dogs and their modifications by beta-adrenoceptor blocking drugs. Am Heart J 86:347–358, 1973.
12. Bruyneel KJJ, Opie LH: The value of warning arrhythmias in the prediction of ventricular fibrillation within one hour of coronary occlusion. Experimental studies in the baboon. Am Heart J 86:373–384, 1973.
13. Lie KI, Wellens HJJ, Downar E, Durrer D: Observations on patients with primary ventricular fibrillation complicating acute myocardial infarction. Circulation 52:755–759, 1975.
14. El-Sherif N, Myerburg RJ, Scherlag BJ, Befeler B, Aranda JM, Castellanos A, Lazzara R: Electrocardiographic antecedents of primary ventricular fibrillation. Value of the R-on-T phenomenon in myocardial infarction. Br Heart J 38:415–422, 1976.
15. Wiggers CJ: The mechanism and nature of ventricular fibrillation. Am Heart J 20:399–412, 1940.

16. Wiggers CJ, Wegria R: Ventricular fibrillation due to single, localized induction and condenser shocks applied during the vulnerable phase of ventricular systole. Am J Physiol 128:500–505, 1940.
17. Smirk FH, Palmer DG: A myocardial syndrome: with particular reference to the occurrence of sudden death and of premature systoles interrupting antecedent T waves. Am J Cardiol 6:620–629, 1960.
18. Dhurandhar RW, MacMillan RL, Brown KWG: Primary ventricular fibrillation complicating acute myocardial infarction. Am J Cardiol 27:347–351, 1971.
19. Engel TR, Meister SG, Frankl WS: The 'R-on-T' phenomenon. An update and critical review. Ann Int. Med 88:221–225, 1978.
20. Williams DO, Scherlag BJ, Hope RR, El-Sherif N, Lazzara R: The pathophysiology of malignant ventricular arrhythmias during acute myocardial ischemia. Circulation 50:1163–1172, 1974.
21. Klein RC, Vera Z, Mason DT, DeMaria AN, Awan NA, Amsterdam EA: Ambulatory Holter monitor documentation of ventricular tachyarrhythmias as mechanism of sudden death in patients with coronary artery disease. Clin Res 27:7A, 1979. (Abstract.)
22. Liberthson RR, Nagel EL, Hirschman JC, Nussenfeld SR, Blackbourne BD, Davis JH: Pathophysiologic observations in prehospital ventricular fibrillation and sudden cardiac death. Circulation 49:790–798, 1974.
23. Baum RS, Alvarez H III, Cobb LA: Survival after resuscitation from out-of-hospital ventricular fibrillation. Circulation 50: 1231–1235, 1974.
24. Lie KI, Wellens HJ, Durrer D: Characteristics and predictability of primary ventricular fibrillation. Eur J Cardiol 1/4:379–384, 1974.
25. Adgey AAJ, Nelson PG, Scott ME, Geddes JS, Allen JD, Zaidi SA, Pantridge JF: Management of ventricular fibrillation outside hospital. Lancet 1:1169–1171, 1969.
26. Adgey AAJ, Devlin JE, Webb SW, Mulholland HC: Initiation of ventricular fibrillation outside hospital in patients with acute ischaemic heart disease. Br Heart J 47:55–61, 1982.

5. BIOMEDICAL ENGINEERING IN MOBILE CORONARY CARE

John Anderson*

1. INTRODUCTION

Mobile coronary care was established by Pantridge and Geddes in 1966 [1]. It utilized a mains-operated DC defibrillator powered by a static inverter which converted a 12V car battery supply to 230V (Figure 1). The total package weighed approximately 110 lbs and although extremely cumbersome, allowed defibrillation to take place outside the hospital for the first time. A Cambridge recorder provided monitoring of the patient's electrocardiogram. It was also battery-operated. The equipment was unsuitable for the intended environment in that it was heavy, consumed considerable power and was not purpose-designed. The engineering possibilities were obvious. Lightweight defibrillators with internal battery supplies and suitable monitoring systems were required if mobile coronary care was to become widespread.

The early engineering approach to mobile coronary care in Belfast was to design portable instruments to fulfil the necessary medical requirements. These were carried in a standard-type ambulance with minimal modifications to its structure. The American Optical company was approached in 1968 and produced the first entirely portable DC defibrillator weighing approximately 44 lbs (Figure 2). The defibrillator was powered by a 28V mercury cell battery pack and provided approximately 100 shots of 400 W-s stored energy. The unit also contained a 'back-up' supply which could be immediately accessed via a front panel switch. The circuit design was fairly simple, consisting of a power oscillator supplying a long and inefficient multiplier chain which provided 7 kV to a 16 μf storage capacitor. The energy was switched via a single pole sealed vacuum relay, the other terminal of the capacitor being referred to the ground paddle. The choke value at 100 mH produced the Lown waveform and delivered approximately 270 W-s into a 50 Ω load. The monitoring system as shown in Figure 3 consisted of a Cardiostat T (Siemens) electrocardiographic recorder and an Elema Schonander 3" display oscilloscope which were bolted together to provide a complete recording system. The instrument could provide continuous monitoring for up to 6 h and produce a full-lead selection writeout of the electrocardiogram. For the first time now it was relatively easy to monitor the patient at the site of the attack and to continue monitoring until arrival at the hospital coronary care unit.

* Mr. John Anderson was formerly Head of Biomedical Engineering at the Regional Medical Cardiology Centre for Northern Ireland.

Adgey, AAJ (ed): Acute phase of ischemic heart disease and myocardial infarction.
© *1982, Martinus Nijhoff, The Hague, Boston, London. ISBN-13: 978-94-009-7581-1*

78

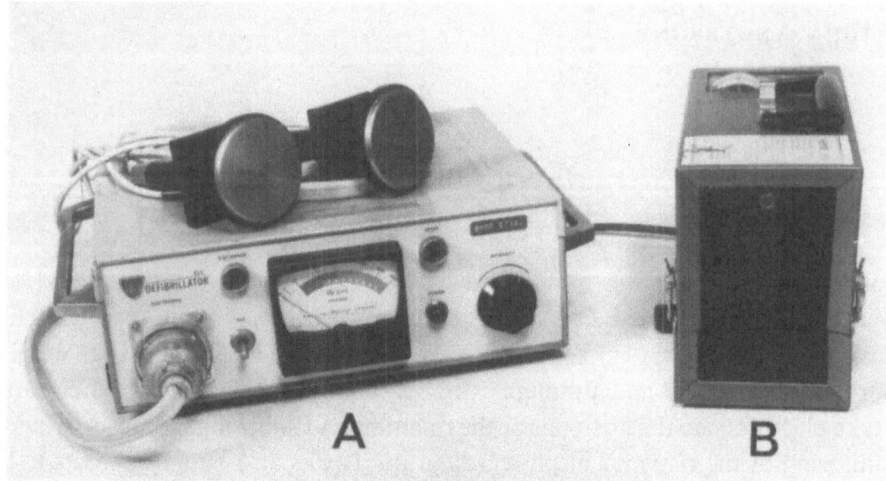

Figure 1. Mains-operated defibrillator and static inverter.
A. Mains-operated defibrillator
B. Static Inverter

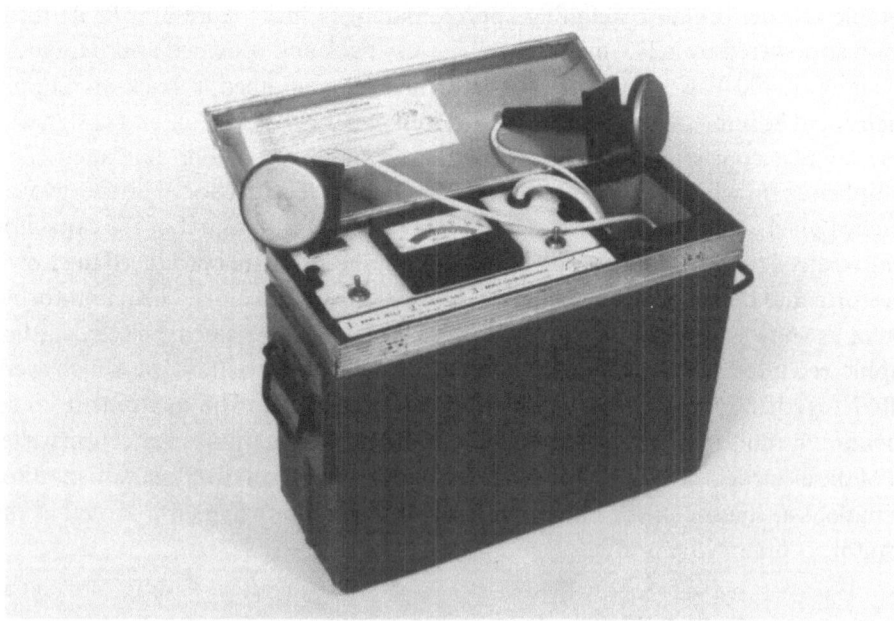

Figure 2. American Optical Portable Defibrillator.

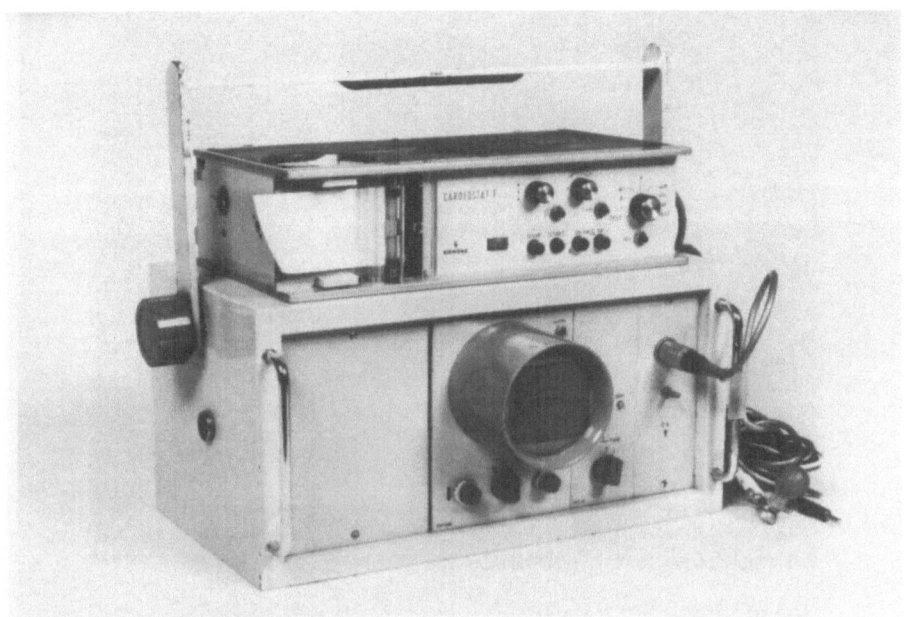

Figure 3. Elema Schonander monitoring and Siemens Cardiostat T recording apparatus.

2. DC DEFIBRILLATOR DEVELOPMENT

The single heaviest piece of equipment was still the defibrillator and design parameters were established to consider the engineering possibilities of reducing the
overall weight without decreasing the effectiveness of the device.

2.1. Design parameters

- Weight: to be considerably less than the American Optical unit
- Portability
- Battery-operated with replaceable and rechargeable batteries
- Reasonable charge time, i.e. 10 s or less to 400 W-s stored
- Delivery: at least 30 shots of 400 W-s stored energy
- Necessary safety requirements
- An effective waveform with the required delivered energy

The specification was general but since the majority of the parameters mentioned
were affected in some way by the main storage device, i.e. the capacitor, it was
decided to begin the investigation at this point. The Lown waveform did not lend
itself easily to a battery-operated portable device. The high voltages required i.e.,
7 kV to charge a 16 μf capacitor to 400 W-s stored, led to a number of design
difficulties. The capacitor required high voltage dielectric material, the charging

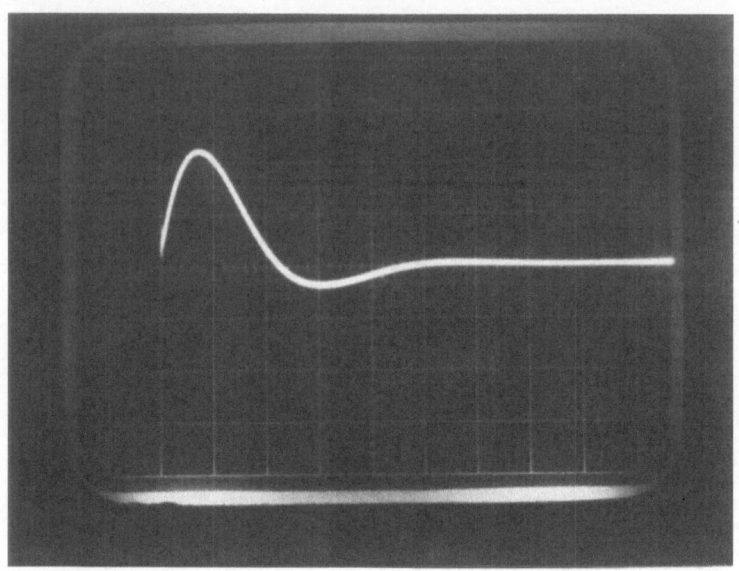

Figure 4. 'Lown' Waveform.
Timebase   – 2 ms/cm
External Load   – 50 Ω

circuits (traditionally voltage multipliers) were inefficient and the delivered energy was reduced because the high source current increased the losses in the output circuitry, i.e. only 270 W-s delivered into 50 Ω from a stored energy of 400 W-s.

2.1.1. Waveform optimisation

A major design consideration was to optimise a waveform which would allow maximum weight reduction of the instrument yet retain the capability of being at least as effective as the Lown format.

Lown [2] who described the Lown waveform did not clearly indicate the reasons for the selection of this particular wave shape. It appeared similar to the shape of an AC waveform (i.e. $\frac{1}{2}$ sine wave) with a similar amount of energy as that traditionally delivered by an AC defibrillator. The following are the characteristics of AC defibrillation:

- frequency: 60 Hz
- voltage range: 150–750V
- time: 150 ms

Energy generated by AC waveform assuming a 50 Ω load

$$= V \times I \times t \text{ W-s}$$

$$\text{If } V = 150 \text{ volts } I = \frac{150}{50} = 3 \text{ Amps}$$

$$\text{W-s} = 150 \times 3 \times .15 \simeq 70 \text{ W-s}$$

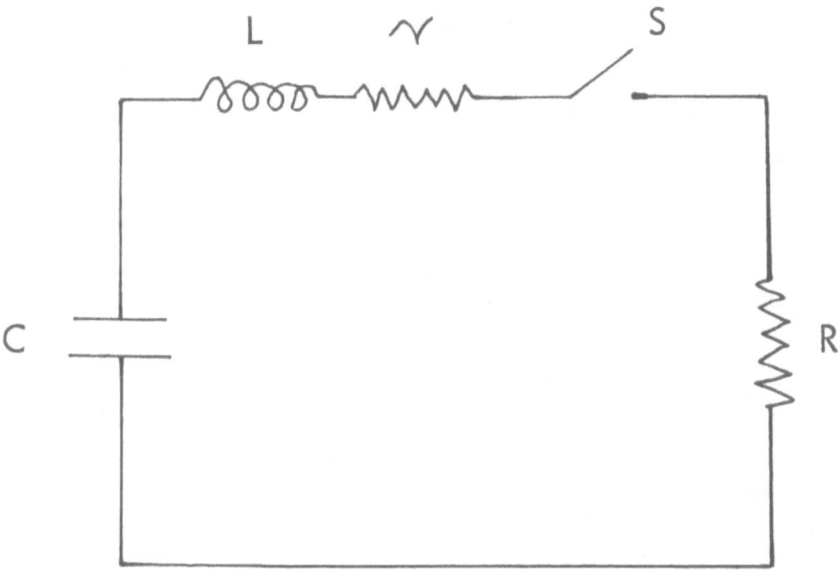

Figure 5. Simplified discharge network.

C – storage capacitor	S – high voltage switch
L – inductor	R – external load
r – internal resistance of inductor	R + r = R′ = total circuit resistance

$$\text{If V} = 750 \text{ volts } I = \frac{750}{50} = 15 \text{ Amps}$$

$$\text{W-s} = 750 \times 15 \times .15 \simeq 1700 \text{ W-s}$$

Zoll et al. [3] using an AC defibrillator reported that optimal values for conversion appeared to lie between 240 and 360 volts, i.e. an average energy around 250 W-s. It would appear that Lown effectively reproduced a similar amount of stored energy and delivered it in a half sine wave format. This required him to charge a 16 μf capacitor to 7 kV and discharge the energy through a 100 mH, 20 Ω choke producing the well-known Lown waveform [2]. The performance of this DC waveform was evaluated in animal studies, and indicated that the discharge was more effective and less likely to cause arrhythmias than an AC discharge. Figure 4 shows the discharge characteristics of the Lown waveform. The instrument was discharged into a 50 Ω load and the time-base is displayed at 2 ms/cm. However, as already mentioned this waveform because of its high voltage requirement and output losses, was not the most suitable for the development of a miniature defibrillator.

Any new waveform requires a number of specifications, i.e. voltage amplitude, damping factor, pulse width, etc., but the essential difference in our development was that the different wave shapes theoretically produced were compared with the actual weight of the components used to generate them. The discharge system may be treated as a simple R,L,C circuit as shown in Figure 5. The circuit behaves as follows: when switch S is closed the initial current is represented by

$$-\frac{1}{C}\int i\,dt = L\frac{di}{dt} + R'i$$

differentiating $-\dfrac{i}{C} = L\dfrac{d^2i}{dt^2} + R'\dfrac{di}{dt}$

or $(D^2 + \dfrac{R'}{L}D + \dfrac{1}{LC})\ i = 0$

taking roots $D_1 = \dfrac{-\dfrac{R'}{L} + \sqrt{\dfrac{(R')^2}{(L)} - \dfrac{4}{LC}}}{2} = \alpha + \beta$

and $D_2 = \dfrac{-\dfrac{R'}{L} - \sqrt{\dfrac{(R')^2}{(L)} - \dfrac{4}{LC}}}{2} = \alpha - \beta$

while $\alpha = -\dfrac{R'}{2L}$, $\beta = \sqrt{\dfrac{(R')^2}{(2L)} - \dfrac{1}{LC}}$

Three conditions may now be represented.

Condition (i) $\dfrac{(R')^2}{(2L)} > \dfrac{1}{LC}$

This condition represents the overdamped transient.

$\{D - (\alpha + \beta)\}\ \{D - (\alpha - \beta)\}\ i\,(t) = 0$
$i\,(t) = C_1\,e^{(\alpha + \beta)t} + C_2\,e^{(\alpha - \beta)t}$

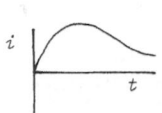

Condition (ii) $\dfrac{(R')^2}{(2L)} = \dfrac{1}{LC}$

critically damped waveform

$\beta = 0\quad (D - \alpha)^2\ i = 0$
Therefore $i(t) = e^{\alpha t}\,(C_1 + C_2\,t)$

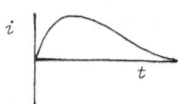

Condition (iii) $\dfrac{(R')^2}{(2L)} < \dfrac{1}{LC}$

oscillatory decay

$\beta = \sqrt{\dfrac{1}{LC} - \dfrac{(R')^2}{(2L)}}$

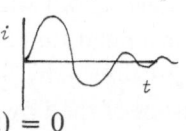

Therefore $\{D - (\alpha + j\beta)\}\ \{D - (\alpha - j\beta)\}\ i(t) = 0$
$i(t) = e^{\alpha t}\,(C_1\,\cos\beta t + C_2\,\sin\beta t)$

It can therefore be seen that the three expressions defined represent the discharge characteristics of the R,L,C circuit. Using the formulae demonstrated, a computer program was constructed into which a wide range of variables were fed. These variables were:
- Stored energy: 400 W-s
- Capacitance range: 8–100 μf

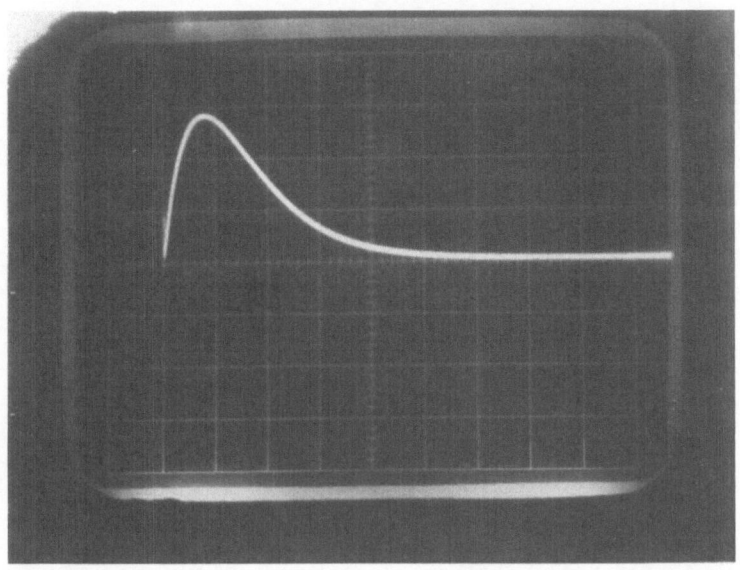

Figure 6. 'Pantridge' Waveform.
Timebase   – 2 ms/cm
External Load   – 50 Ω

- Inductor range: 10–100 mH
- Inductor impedance: 3–50 Ω
- Load resistance: 50 Ω

The program was instructed to select those values which would produce a waveform between $2\frac{1}{2}$ and 6 ms measured at the $\frac{1}{2}$ power point. The voltage range was determined as not less than 2 kV and not more than 7 kV. Various waveforms were then plotted from the computer results and compared with the weight of the components necessary to generate them. This further analysis produced values of 50 mH, 50 μf for the capacitor, between 14 and 20 Ω for the internal resistance of the inductor, with the discharge characteristics as shown in Figure 6 ('Pantridge' waveform) [4].

The engineering analysis was now complete but the waveform had to be proved effective in the removal of ventricular fibrillation. A series of experiments were conducted in the dog laboratory and it was shown that the waveform was at least as effective as the Lown format at 400 W-s stored, and appeared to be more successful at lower energies.

The first instrument produced using the 'Pantridge' waveform weighed approximately 15 lbs and was code named the Pantridge Portable 15 (Figure 7). The device was manufactured under licence by the Coleraine Instrument Company and had the following specification:

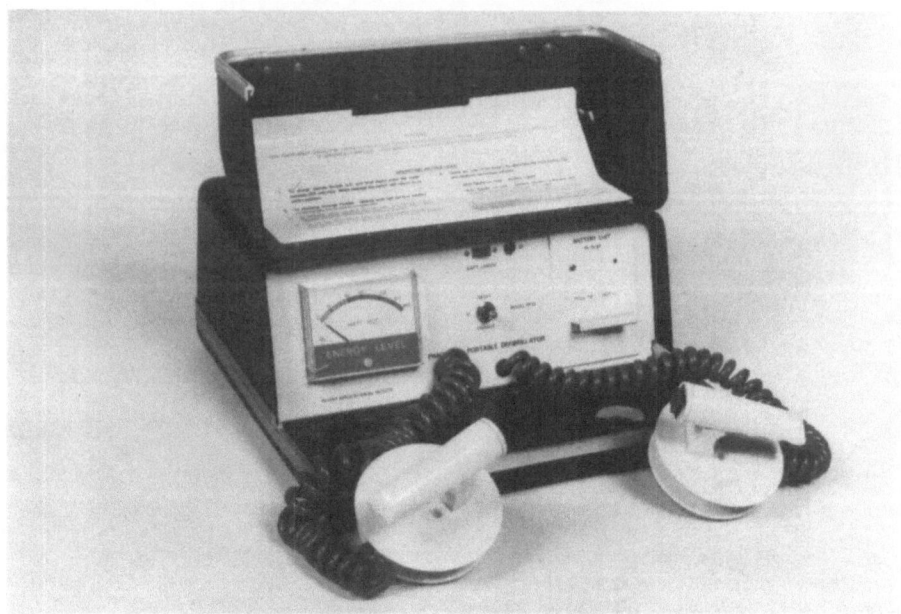

Figure 7. Pantridge Portable 15 Defibrillator.

Power	– Replaceable 20.4V rechargeable nickel-cadmium battery with 1.2 ampere hour capacity sufficient for at least 70 shocks
Energy range	– Stored energy adjustable from 0–400 W-s; maximum delivered energy into 50 Ω load - 330 W-s
Pulse width	– 12–16 ms (critically damped into 50 Ω load)
Pulse rise time	– 1100 μs
Charge time	– 8 s (to 400 W-s stored from fully charged battery)
Weight	– approximately 15 lbs
Control	– A single 3 position switch provides all control functions; an internal bank of resistors is provided for discharging unwanted energy
Capacitor	– 50 μf, 4 kV electrolytic capacitor manufactured by Plessey

The instrument was first manufactured in 1971 and became standard mobile coronary care equipment during this period. Particular attractions were the low weight, simple controls and replaceable battery function. The instrument continued to be manufactured until 1974 and proved to be very reliable.

3. MONITORING DEVELOPMENTS

In 1973 an additional requirement was requested of the engineering staff. A study

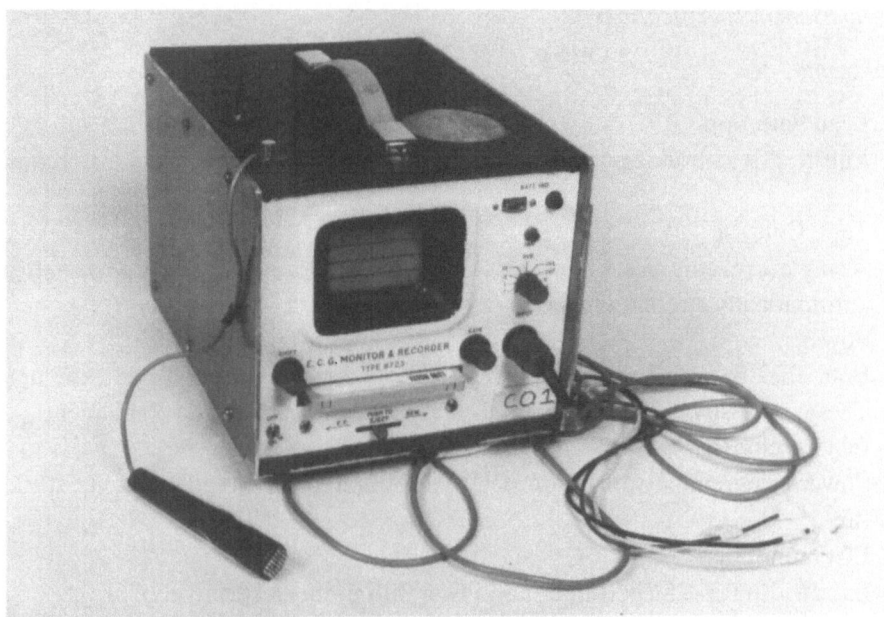

Figure 8. Combined oscilloscope and recording apparatus (C.O.R.A.)

was to be introduced in the out-of-hospital environment which required not only continuous electrocardiographic monitoring of the patient at the site of the attack and until the arrival in the hospital coronary care unit, but also a permanent record which was easily accessible for recall purposes. The combination of the Elema Schonander scope and Siemens write-out (Figure 3) although performing a basic operation contained no easily accessible means of recording a continuous and permanent record of all events. A new design specification for portable monitoring with permanent recording was drafted.

3.1. Instrument requirements

- Lightweight
- Battery-operated
- Continuous visual monitoring
- Replaceable batteries
- Full-lead selection
- Permanent and continuous recording for future analysis

A system was developed encompassing the six basic requirements. The display system was based on a 3″ Telefunken electrostatic oscilloscope tube combined with a front loading cassette tape deck for recording purposes. The unit (Figure 8) became affectionately known as C.O.R.A. (Combined oscilloscope and recording apparatus).

3.2. Instrument specifications

Display unit

- Lead Selection
  Full-lead selection is provided with automatic blocking between switch positions.
- Tape Control
  A single level controls manual ejection of the tape cassette. The tape cassette is automatically ejected when end of run is reached.
- Power
  Four PP9 batteries provide power for both the oscilloscope and tape unit. These are easily accessible through a panel at the back of the instrument.
- ECG oscilloscope
  Power requirement was minimised by the choice of a directly heated cathode tube.
- ECG amplifier
  Bandwidth 0.1–75 Hz (upper and lower 3db points respectively).
- C.M.R.R. (common mode rejection ratio)
  In excess of 85 db, with 5 k Ω in balance.

Tape system

Two channels are provided by means of a special recording head. The first channel utilises pulse-width modulation of the electrocardiographic signal to provide best conditions in terms of Wow and Flutter. The second track is a speech channel, and this is DC biased to minimise cross talk between the speech and electrocardiographic tracks. Figure of merit is better than 45 dB and the tape bandwidth - 8 kHz better than 12 dB on 1 kHz. Up to one hour's information can be stored on a single cassette tape.

Tape Head characteristics

- No. 1 Track (ECG)
- 76 mH. 121 Ω d.c. output – 600 microvolts.
- No. 2 Track (speech)
- 52mH. 95 Ω d.c. output – 220 microvolts.
- Bias current @ 50 kHz – 52 μA
- Record current – 72 μA

Deck

- Wow and Flutter – $\pm$ 0.2% max
- Rumble – 53 dB

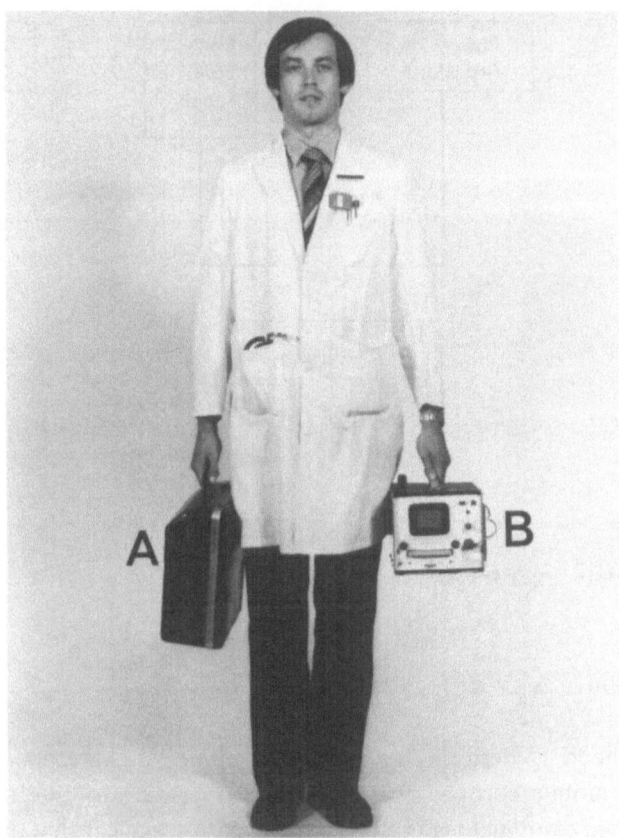

Figure 9. Defibrillator and recording apparatus carried by medical staff.
A. PP15 Defibrillator
B. Combined oscilloscope and recording apparatus

This lightweight portable monitoring facility allowed not only continuous monitoring of the patient's data outside hospital but also easy access for recall purposes.
The tape recording facility provided a complete record of the electrocardiogram,
and the second track, a speech channel, for on-the-spot comments on changes in
blood pressure, injection of drugs, movement of patient etc.

A fast-scan recovery system was also designed and built, enabling the one-hour
tape to be scanned in five minutes. The scan could at any time be stopped and
permanent hard copies of the electrocardiogram with any corresponding speech
comments documented for further comment by the medical staff.

This portable monitoring facility had three major advantages in that the weight of
the apparatus was significantly reduced, continuous recording of all relevant data
was achieved and tapes were reusable when analysis was complete. Three combined
oscilloscope and recording apparatuses were constructed and have been in constant
use for seven years, providing a data bank of ambulatory information.

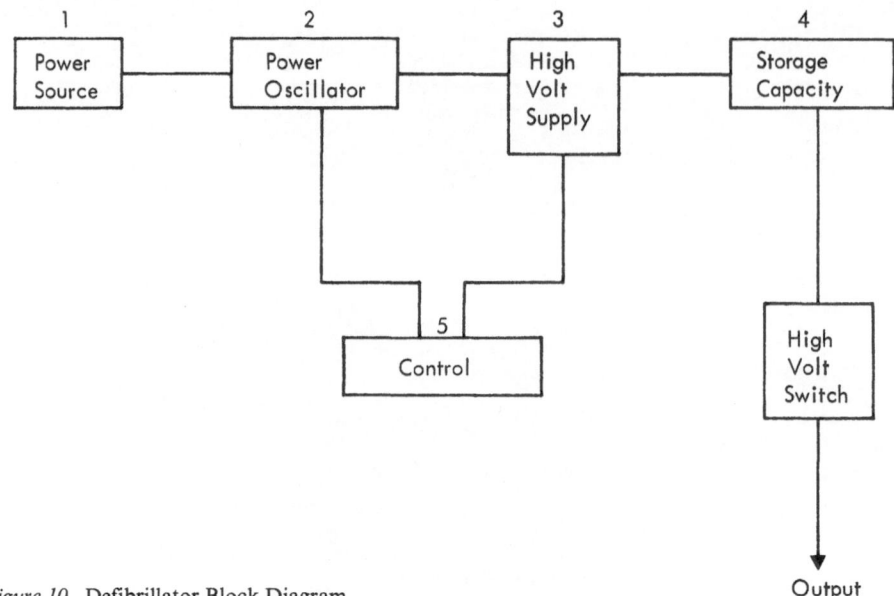

Figure 10. Defibrillator Block Diagram.

4. MOBILE CORONARY CARE SYSTEM

In 1974 with the PP15 defibrillator and the combined oscilloscope and recording apparatus the mobile coronary care unit was operating for the first time with purpose-designed equipment (Figure 9). However, it was clear that the defibrillator with its bulk and weight required further development.

5. FURTHER DEFIBRILLATOR DEVELOPMENTS

A defibrillator may be represented by a number of building blocks (Figure 10). The main contributors to component weight in defibrillator instruments are found in sections 1 and 4 and although sections 2, 3 and 5 tend to provide the bulk of the circuitry they do not seriously affect the overall weight (Figure 10). However if the efficiency of the charging circuit is improved, the battery size can be reduced, i.e. the same number of shots can be obtained from a smaller power source. The single most significant weight contributor was the capacitor at 2.8 lbs and the next design phase of our defibrillator development would have been largely ineffective, unless this component could have been greatly reduced.

5.1. Kureha KF film developments

In 1971 during component sourcing contact was made with Capacitor Specialists Incorporated of Escondido, Calif. At that time this company was manufacturing

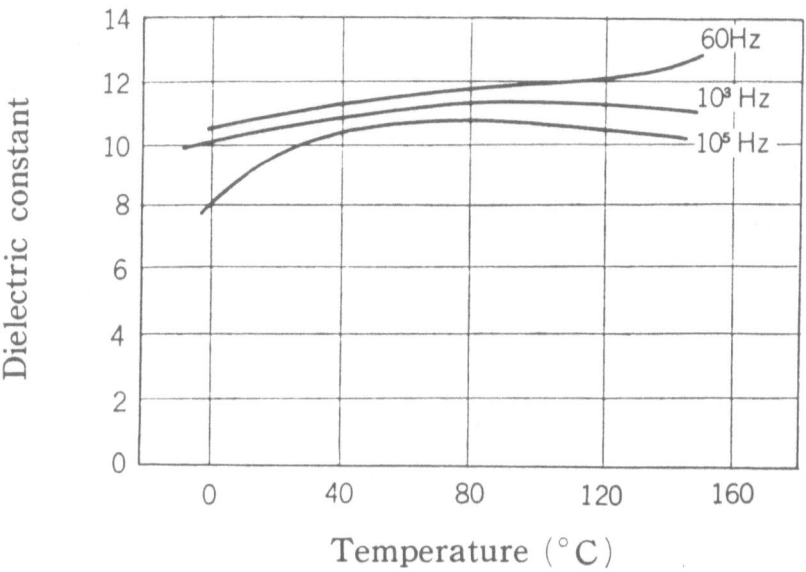

Figure 11. Electrical properties of Kureha KF Film – dielectric constant and temperature.

most of the standard mylar type capacitors for defibrillators. Further discussions on methods of reducing capacitor size revealed a new material Kureha KF film which it was thought might provide the vehicle for the development of much lighter capacitors. Kureha KF film has a number of advantages along with a dielectric constant almost 3 times that of mylar.

General properties of Kureha KF film

- – Highest dielectric constant in plastic film
- – Mechanically very tough
- – Non-flammable
- – Good thermal stability
- – Excellent weathering resistance and good stability to ultraviolet rays and radiation
- – Excellent resistance to insulation oils and almost all chemicals
- – Low water absorption
- – Low gas permeability
- – No plasticizers are required

Figures 11, 12 and 13 show the general electrical properties of Kureha KF film. It required several years of intensive development before the first K film series

* K film is a registered trade mark of CSI Kureha KF film capacitors.

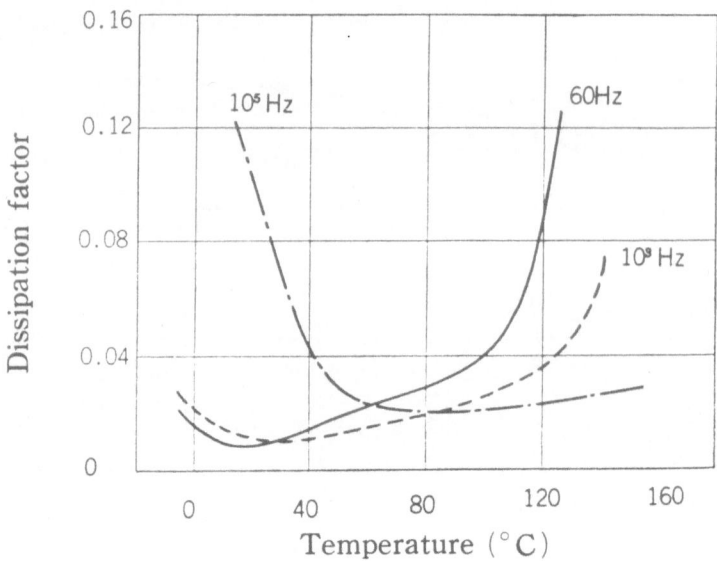

Figure 12. Electrical properties of Kureha KF Film – dissipation factor and temperature.

capacitors became available*. A large number of units were cycled and a constant failure analysis was provided before the appropriate acquired quality levels were established. Eventually the unit was developed where it could be used in a defibrillator and became one of the major factors in the reduction of weight and size of defibrillators. Figure 14 shows a standard mylar film capacitor (A) against the first K film unit (B) and a further development (C) which was ultimately used in the Pantridge 6 series defibrillator.

5.2. Other circuitry

The power oscillator unit was reduced in size and the multiplier length optimised. New high energy density nickel cadmium cells were tested and a smaller discharge relay sourced. During the weighing of the various components including the paddles, it was noticed that the total volume of the various pieces sitting on the scales with the paddle underneath might be altered by a completely new concept. This development became a patented feature known as 'electronics within one or both paddles' and has remained a major feature of all our defibrillator developments.

The first defibrillator incorporating these new developments was hand-constructed in the electronic laboratories of the Royal Victoria Hospital, Belfast and was evaluated in 1974. In 1975, Cardiac Recorders of London began manufacture of the 280 series defibrillator (Figure 15) which was based on the original development in the Royal Victoria Hospital, Belfast. The unit proved very popular and had the following specification:

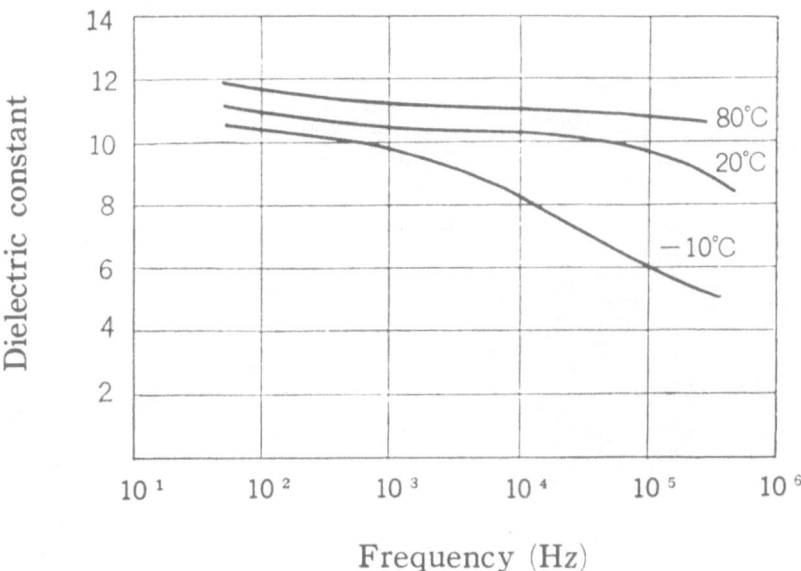

Figure 13. Electrical properties of Kureha KF Film – dielectric constant and frequency.

- Waveform – as described
- Delivered energy per shock – maximum 320 W-s from 400 W-s stored
- Storage capacitor – PVdF type approx 46 μf
- Normal charging voltage – 4200 V
- Paddle size – 85 mm dia
- Analog meter displaying stored energy 0–400 J, and delivered energy 0–320 J (into 50 Ω)
- Control on case – push button ON/OFF switch with built-in battery indicator lights; Push button charge/discharge switch
- Control on paddles, push buttons – defibrillator switch (both switches must be depressed for discharge to occur)
- Size – 13″ long x 4$\frac{1}{4}$″ wide x 7$\frac{1}{2}$″ high
- Weight – 7.5 lbs
- Housing material – injection moulded case from ABS plastic

The unit was at that time at least half the weight of its nearest competitor. The simple controls meant easy operation in the emergency situation. A significant safety feature was the removal of possible external leakage paths between the operator and the patient. As the unit could be left on continuous charge it meant that the unit could be charged rapidly when required and could also be checked at regular intervals. For the first time, a really lightweight purpose designed defibrillator was available.

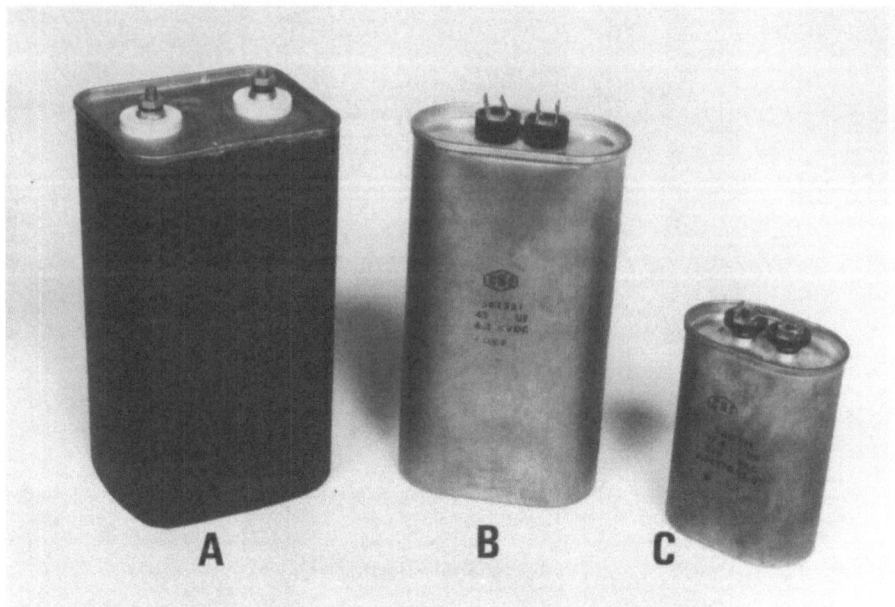

Figure 14. Mylar Film capacitor and Kureha KF Film capacitors.
A: Mylar film capacitor
B and C: Kureha KF film capacitors

6. ON-GOING DEVELOPMENT COMBINING MONITOR WITH DEFIBRILLATOR

The 280 series defibrillator required the addition of an electrocardiographic monitor and considerations were given in 1974 to the development of a combined system. It was possible to produce a unit with the traditional oscilloscopic tube and a number of different prototypes were considered. However, a combination of the capacitor size and the length of the display tubes as a ratio of the viewing area made it difficult to design an optimal system. Flat screen displays were considered as an alternative for producing a combined defibrillator monitor.

6.1. Techniques for presenting data on a flat screen

There are a variety of methods which might allow data to be presented on a flat screen. It was decided to investigate the following in an attempt to ascertain the most suitable materials: plasma matrix, liquid crystal, light-emitting diodes, electro-optic, and electroluminescent. A number of plasma matrix formats were investigated including the self-scan type. However, it was not possible to achieve sufficient line density to make this type of structure suitable for the display of an electro-cardiogram. Liquid crystal displays were attractive for two reasons:

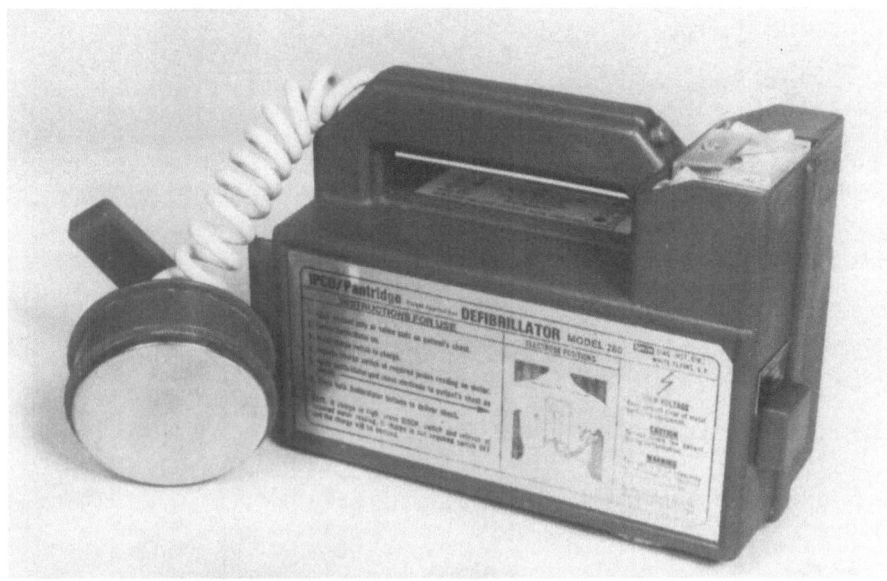

Figure 15. Cardiac recorders 280 series Pantridge defibrillator.

1) They have the ability to display data in bright sunlight
2) They do not require the high drive voltages necessary for many other flat screen displays

However, even if the 'bright-up display' technique (information presented as a refresh display from a buffer memory) was not used and information was displayed in real time, i.e. 1 frame/s, it would require a liquid crystal switching time of 200 ms at $-15°$ C. This is currently not possible and portable displays would have to be pre-heated to around 20° C to guarantee reasonable performance. Thus, although liquid crystal displays should not be entirely ruled out their application in the mobile environment was not considered practical. The large light-emitting diode display is presently at a crossroads between monolithic and discrete assembly. The former approach is more limited by high power dissipation and non-uniform yield, whereas the latter is rather limited in resolution and fabrication cost. In addition there are still problems associated with low luminous efficiency, differential ageing, and high power consumption which limit light-emitting diode displays in the large display domain. There are a number of electro-optic displays other than the basic liquid crystal. Yet, most structures require the movement of particles as the mechanism of light modulation. The present response time of such structures is approximately 10 ms at 15 v. The devices tend to remain in the last driver state, i.e. particles-up or particles-down, and the cell structure requires a 'driver off' as well as a 'driver on' condition. In particular, the life cycles tend to be only in the order of 3000 h. It is unlikely that this type of structure will ever be suitable for real-time information display.

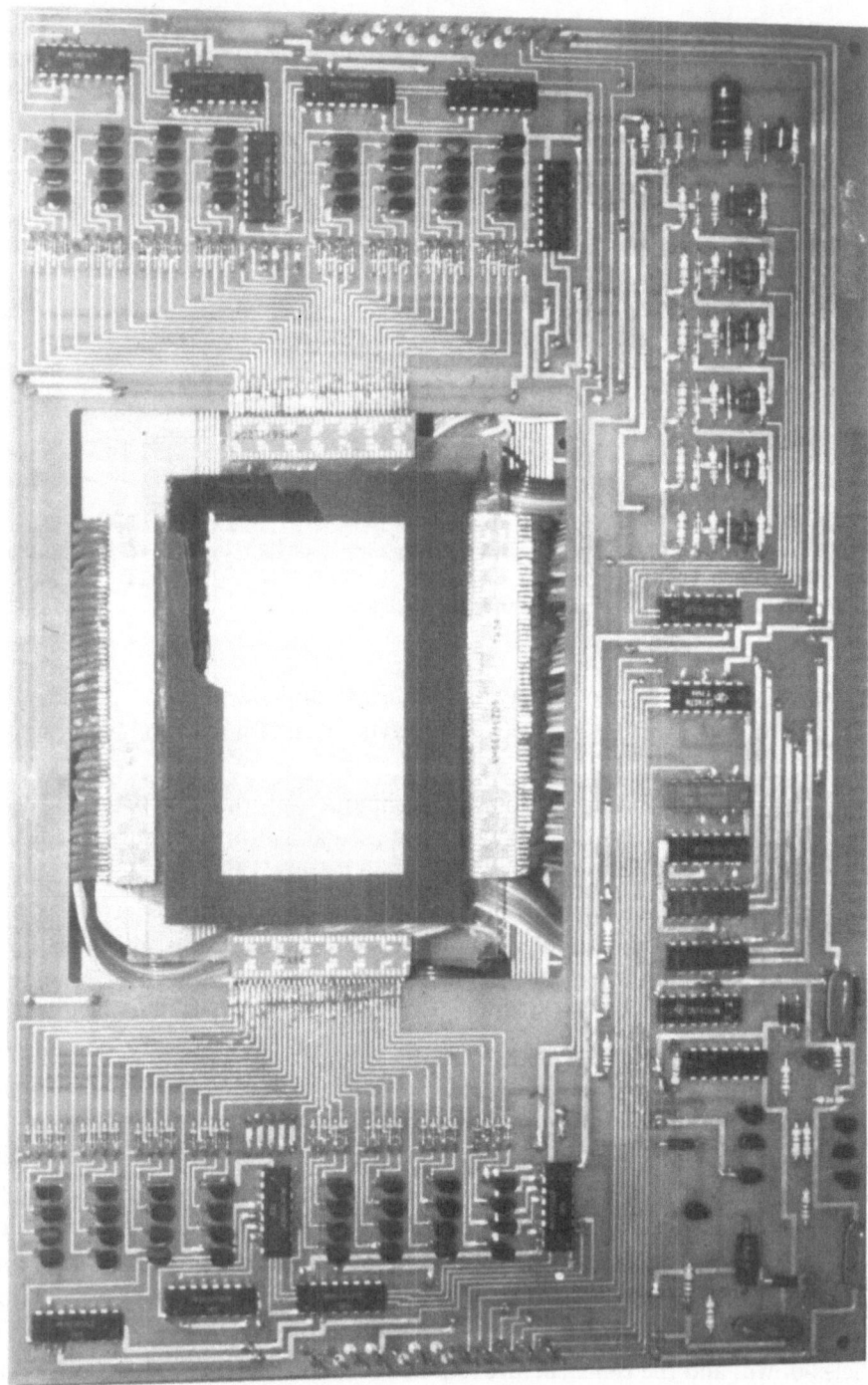

Figure 16. Prototype electroluminescent display.

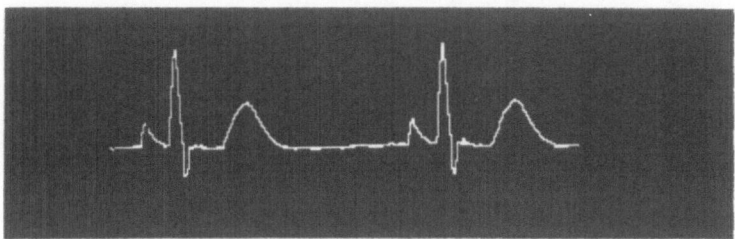

Figure 17. Sinus rhythm on a flat screen format.

Electroluminescent displays, apart from the driving technology appear to offer the most costeffective method of developing a dense matrix suitable for the display of information in a flat plane. The fabrication of such panels is a relatively simple process employing the use of basic silk-screen technology and mechanical scribing. A prototype unit was designed and constructed to evaluate the possibility of displaying an electrocardiogram on a dot matrix structure. Figure 16 shows a prototype electroluminescent panel with a line resolution of 80 per inch. Figures 17 and 18 show sinus rhythm and ventricular fibrillation displayed on a flat screen format. Special driving technology was developed to produce an interpolated display to 'fill-in' between the dots. These techniques combined with a line density of 80 lines/inch produced an acceptable picture which clearly distinguishes between lethal and non-lethal dysrhythmias.

However, a further development program must be completed to optimise the drive circuitry before this type of display could be utilized within the limitations of a portable defibrillator.

7. ON-GOING DEFIBRILLATOR DEVELOPMENT

The reduction in defibrillator size has continued. The current unit manufactured in Northern Ireland weighs only 6½ lbs (Figure 19) and utilises a capacitor similar to that shown in Figure 14 (C). Future development in capacitors particularly with regard to the use of metalisation technology, should see the development of a 3-4 lb

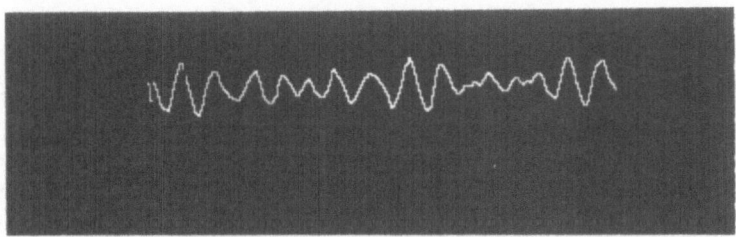

Figure 18. Ventricular fibrillation on a flat screen format.

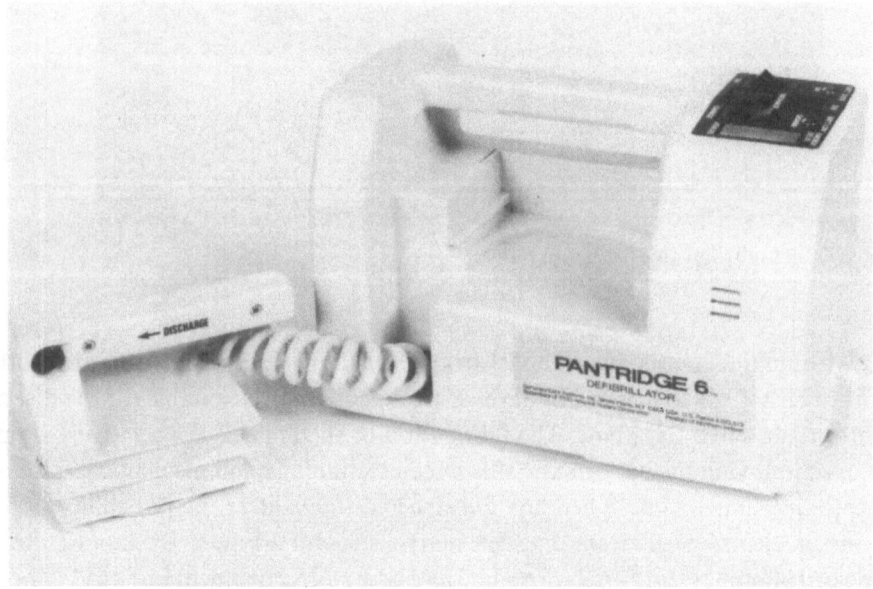

Figure 19. Pantridge portable defibrillator Model PP6.

pocket defibrillator within the next 5 years. It is intended that these small lightweight defibrillators are made available to trained personnel for use outside hospital. However, the general population could not be trained in sufficient numbers and to the level required where the decision to defibrillate is placed in their hands. Software has been developed at the Cardiology Department of the Royal Victoria Hospital, Belfast which can, without the aid of a learning beat and in the presence of significant artifact clearly detect ventricular fibrillation from other dysrhythmias. Hopefully, within the next few years units will be developed with pattern recognition capabilities included in the defibrillator enabling for the first time defibrillation to become as easily available as cardiopulmonary resuscitation.

8. CONCLUSIONS

Mobile coronary care has become an integral part of the practice of medicine. Engineering support has enabled developments to take place which have produced custom made instruments for out-of-hospital coronary care. Future developments such as flat screen displays, miniaturised capacitors and pattern recognition defibrillators promise a great increase in the practice of this type of emergency medicine. Hopefully this dynamic approach to critical care medicine will greatly reduce many of the unfortunate early and very often unnecessary sudden deaths.

REFERENCES

1. Pantridge JF, Geddes JS: Cardiac arrest after myocardial infarction. Lancet 1:807–808, 1966.
2. Lown B, Neuman J, Amarasingham R, Berkovits BV: Comparison of alternating current with direct electroshock across the closed chest. Am J Cardiol 10:223–233, 1962.
3. Zoll PM, Paul MH, Linenthal AJ, Norman LR, Gibson W: Effects of external electric currents on heart: control of cardiac rhythm and induction and termination of cardiac arrhythmias. Circulation 14:745–756, 1956.
4. Pantridge JF, Adgey AAJ, Webb SW, Anderson J: Electrical requirements for ventricular defibrillation. Br Med J 2:313–315, 1975.

6. MOBILE PRE-HOSPITAL CORONARY CARE – COLUMBUS, OHIO

JOHN M. STANG, MARTIN D. KELLER and RICHARD P. LEWIS

1. INTRODUCTION

The City of Columbus, Ohio, USA has a population of approximately 565,000 residing within an area of 184 square miles. It exceeds the population of Denver and Atlanta by at least 50 000 people, and over the past twenty years has grown faster than any other city in the northeastern industrial quadrant of the United States [1]. It is a city constructed on flat terrain with efficient surface transportation related to criss-crossing major arteries in the center of the city and a surrounding 'outerbelt'. The most readily recognizable feature of the city is the Ohio State University, which contributes 54 462 students to the overall population. The Ohio State University Hospital is but one of eight hospitals that are capable of taking care of the coronary patient.

The City of Columbus has enjoyed an efficient pre-hospital rescue system for over fifty years. The City as such was founded in 1834, and it was 100 years later, in 1934, that the Chief of the Division of Fire and two firefighters were called upon to respond personally to a telephone linesman who was a victim of electrocution. The newspaper story which followed made the fire division and the general public aware of the need for a formalized rescue system, and in the same year the now famous Six-Hose Wagon was created, the first 'Squad' under the direction of Chief Edward P. Welch. People then began to call the Fire Department for help in times of crisis, and this habit has continued to the present day.

The first annual Squad Report was collated in 1936, 52 runs being recorded in that early experience. A second Squad was added in 1938, culminating into the establishment of a fleet of seven Squad vehicles by the mid-1960's. It was this pre-hospital system unto which mobile coronary care was grafted.

2. MOBILIZED PRE-HOSPITAL CORONARY CARE – THE FLYING SQUAD OF BELFAST

The 1960's witnessed an extraordinary evolution in the concept of coronary care. In 1962, Day reported his early results with an in-hospital specialized unit designed to permit the prompt recognition of in-hospital infarction-related cardiac arrest [2]. It was duly recognized that the risk of death from myocardial infarction was probably

Adgey, AAJ (ed): Acute phase of ischemic heart disease and myocardial infarction.
© *1982, Martinus Nijhoff, The Hague, Boston, London. ISBN-13: 978-94-009-7581-1*

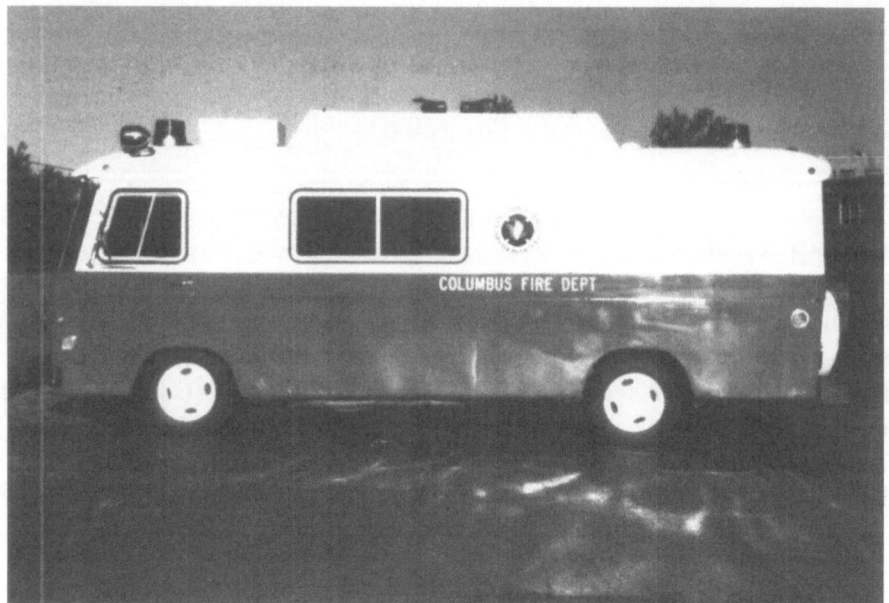

Figure 1. The original Heartmobile® vehicle.

greatest in the first 12 hours following the onset of symptoms, and that many patients died prior to safe transport and admission to the hospital. In response to this problem, a system was devised whereby 'highly mobile units' were used for the treatment of patients with myocardial infarction outside the hospital and for stabilization prior to transportation [3]. These very important early efforts of Pantridge and colleagues in Belfast, Ireland led to the first successful resuscitation from out-of-hospital cardiac arrest [3, 4]. Shortly, thereafter, this concept of pre-hospital mobilized coronary care was transplanted to the United States by the late Dr. William J. Grace in New York City [5], and by Dr. James V. Warren in Columbus [6]. Both systems are still operative and instrumental in the shaping of mobile coronary care in America. The former always fought the gradient created by New York City itself whose very complexity made 'rapid response' virtually impossible.

3. HEARTMOBILE®

During the years 1966 through 1968, there was a long series of intensely emotional and forward-thinking discussions relative to the establishment of pre-hospital resuscitation for victims of myocardial infarction and cardiac arrest in Columbus. In accordance with the expectations there was some degree of reluctance on the part of City officials to embark upon something so unique and novel. By virtue of the courageous and perceptive persistence of Warren, supplemented by the bold determination of safety director James Hughes, the Heartmobile® program was launched.

The Heartmobile® was meant to be a coronary care unit and research laboratory on wheels (Figure 1). It was intended to carry a doctor and specially trained Firefighters, and to be superimposed as a 'second response' vehicle alongside the previously described and pre-existing Squad system. Grants were received from the Regional Medical Programs of the Department of Health Education and Welfare, and the Central Ohio chapter of the American Heart Association (COHA). A volunteer corps of selected Firefighters underwent a twelve-hour course. In October of 1969 the Heartmobile® began operating from the grounds of the Ohio State University Hospital. During these early runs the unit was staffed by members of the Department of Medicine House staff and by Division of Cardiology Post-Doctoral Fellows. This contributed to the relatively slow response time of the original vehicle for, as might be imagined, the relatively large and lumbering vehicle, dispatched from a single central location and perhaps delayed by the summoning of a young doctor otherwise busy on the 11th floor of the hospital, created a relatively inefficient method for rapid pre-hospital response. Telemetry was used during this early experience with the Heartmobile®, transmissions being received on the Coronary Care Unit of the Ohio State University Hospital. The lessons learned from this initial experience between October 1969 and July 1971 were invaluable and may be compared with the subsequent efforts of specially trained Firefighters functioning without the presence of a doctor. The Heartmobile® may be viewed as the vehicle whereby coronary care was gradually eased out of its familiar hospital setting into the streets of Columbus.

4. THE INITIATION OF AUTONOMOUS PROTOCOL-DIRECTED PARAMEDIC
   ACTIVITY – THE MEDIC UNITS WITHIN A MULTI-TIERED
   EMERGENCY MEDICAL SERVICE SYSTEM

The Heartmobile® experience soon indicated a number of important points:
1. Specially trained 'firefighter paramedics' quickly became extraordinarily proficient in medical skills practiced in the context of high volume repeated exposure.
2. It became apparent that telemetry gave rise not only to technical difficulties resulting in frequent delays, but also constituted an artificial barrier to the initiation of resuscitative and therapeutic efforts that were mandated by the particular clinical situation.
3. The presence of a physician in the setting of such pre-hospital scenarios was not often essential as the Firemen themselves quickly learned to function in this narrow and usually brief contact with the patient in a highly competent fashion.
Therefore, in 1971 twenty-two highly experienced firefighter paramedics were selected who had accumulated an average of 2 000 hours of physician-supervised

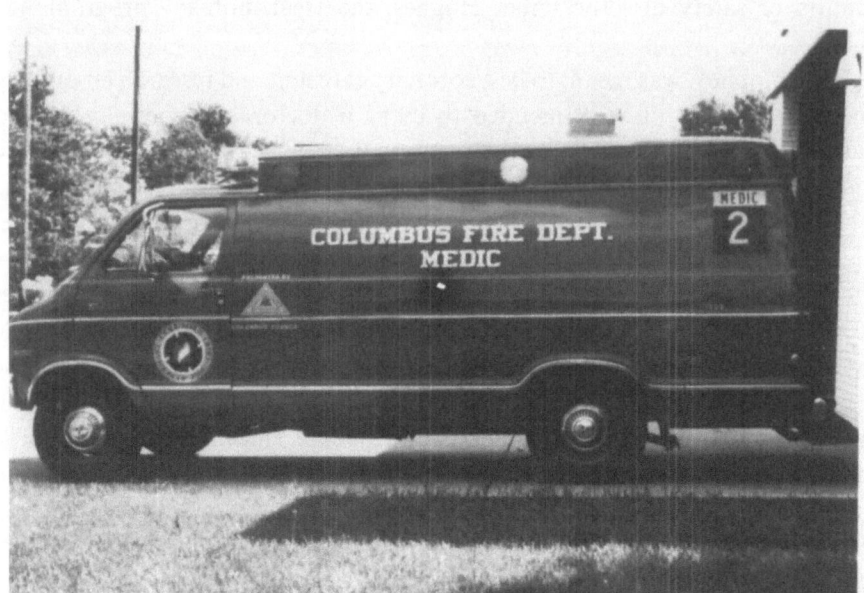

Figure 2. The Medic Vehicle as of 1971.

experience per man. These individuals completed a 64-hour course taught by a physician (RPL) and a newly appointed nurse instructor coordinator, Mrs. Kathryn L. Sampson, BSN. Through gifts from the Horton Ambulance Company, the Columbus Soroptimists, and the Bell Telephone Pioneers, the first of four smaller and more lightweight van-styled Medic Units was purchased (Figure 2). With this preparation, a bold undertaking was initiated on 1 July 1971, viz. an autonomous paramedic activity in Columbus, Ohio. A protocol had been carefully written by physicians from multiple hospitals within the city, and the men were now permitted to act upon their own judgement and as directed by this protocol in the absence of a physician, and this without the use of telemetry. Each of eventually four Medic Vehicles carried three paramedics (EMT-P). As had been true in the past, the Squad vehicles, now numbering seven, each carried two squadmen-paramedics (EMT-A) (Figure 3). In 1973, by the time four Medic units had been established, four Rescue Units were also set up each carrying three firefighters with training equivalent to EMT-A. These men and vehicles were equipped to respond to both fire as well as all complex rescue problems (including extraction of victims pinned, etc.). By this time, the system had become 'multi-tiered', whose four levels of response included the engine companies themselves (all firefighters having been trained in cardio-pulmonary resuscitation), the Rescues, the Squads, and the Medic Units with the most sophisticated vehicles for pre-hospital coronary care as well as for all other types of medical and surgical catastrophe. (Figure 3). Activation of the system was by the citizens, whereby the familiar telephone number of the Fire Department

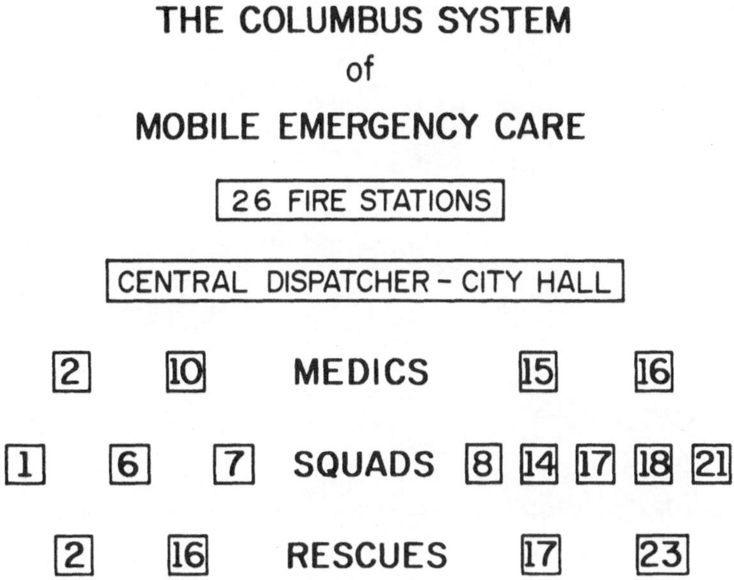

THE COLUMBUS SYSTEM
of
MOBILE EMERGENCY CARE

| 26 FIRE STATIONS |

| CENTRAL DISPATCHER – CITY HALL |

2   10   **MEDICS**   15   16

1   6   7   **SQUADS**   8 14 17 18 21

2   16   **RESCUES**   17   23

Figure 3. A diagrammatic illustration of the structure of the Columbus Emergency Medical Service (EMS) System. The eighth Squad (No. 18) was added one year ago.

could be dialled in case of a perceived cardiac emergency. No charge for this service was made, as the system was supported by City taxes and donations. The cost of operating this system was approximately $ 3.00 per year per tax-paying citizen, a cost which has risen but slightly since then to approximately $ 5.50. The multi-tiered nature of this system provided a rapid response capability, the average response time from moment of calling to arrival of the first vehicle being 3 min. A system of dispatch was developed whereby approximately one dozen cardiac and non-cardiac emergencies prompted the immediate turn-out of one of the four Medics and at least one other vehicle, generally one of the seven Squads (Table 1). Judgement was made by the dispatchers from their interpretation of citizen calls. Depending upon the

Table 1. Perceived pre-hospital emergencies indicating 'double-dispatch' of the nearest Medic plus at least one additional 'first response' vehicle

1. All multi-alarm fires
2. Serious auto accidents
3. Explosions
4. Difficulty in breathing
5. Persons not breathing
6. Chest pains (or any related symptom of heart attack or possible heart attack such as syncope)
7. Shortness of breath
8. Patients pinned (automobile accidents, machinery or cave-ins).
9. Drownings
10. Unconscious patients
11. Electrocutions
12. Any other emergency where the dispatcher feels the Medic Unit may be of service

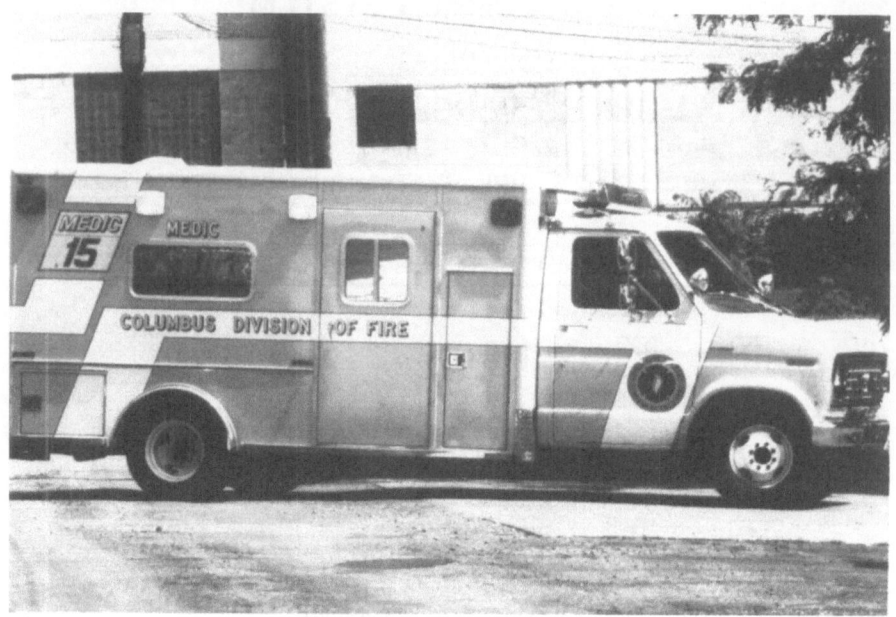

Figure 4. The present day Medic Vehicle.

geographic location of the emergency, the first response vehicle might be one of the four Rescue Units or one of the Ladder Companies. This technique of multi-tiered dispatch provided not only a rapid response, but also a more concentrated experience for the medic personnel as this was one of the ways in which their proficiency and competence was maintained. The current Medic Vehicle is shown in Figure 4.

The multiple levels of responsibility also permit men to become involved in Emergency Medical Service (EMS) work to a degree commensurate with their interest and aptitude. In such a system they are also given the opportunity to vary their experience (by working on various 'tiers') without having to return to pure firefighter status.

The original twenty-two Heartmobile® paramedics provided the basis for the entire system. They themselves and men like them are the experienced 'hands' in the years to follow whereby younger recruits will be trained on the job. This is one of the reasons for the requirement of three paramedics on each Medic vehicle, as such a system guarantees a degree of expertise for every 'run'. By the technique of double dispatch there were at least five individuals at the scene of every victim of cardiac arrest, thus providing more than ample manpower for dealing with the most complex patient. The majority of the original twenty-two paramedics remain within the system now, and continue to provide the type of 'role model' necessary in any such ongoing training program.

5. THE PRESENT STRUCTURE AND FUNCTION OF THE COLUMBUS SYSTEM

The current operation of the Columbus System is very much the kind of system as described above. The Squads see three times as many patients as the Medic Units (Table 2). All patients with suspected acute myocardial infarction, pulmonary edema, and sudden cardiac death in which resuscitation is possible, are handled by the Medic Units working in conjunction with the Squad. The Medic Units transport half of the patients they see, while one-third of those seen by the Squadmen are transported [7] (Table 2). The 'assist' category represents instances in which both units were present. In 14% of instances with the Squads and 29% with the Medics, a run results in no patients seen, the higher figure for the latter reflecting the freedom of the squadmen to 'cancel' the Medic Unit en route when no real emergency is found by the first response team. This technique is used to avoid unnecessary detainment of the fewer Medic Units who are therefore nearly always in a position to respond to the true emergency.

Each Squad makes an average of thirteen runs per day and transports between three and four patients. Each Medic makes an average of ten runs per day and transports three patients. Although Medic involvement with the patient takes considerably more time (with intravenous treatment and other therapeutic interventions), there is roughly an equal distribution of labor. Each Medic Unit sees an average of one victim of myocardial infarction and/or sudden cardiac death per working day. The protocol for chest pain patients is shown in Table 3.

The men are on duty on every third day, for a 24-hour period. Once a week, one unit comes together with the Medical Director and Nurse Coordinator in a 'medic

Table 2. Type of patients seen – annual averages for 1975–1977

Diagnosis	Squad	% of total	Medic	% of total
Neuropsychiatric[a]	2 460	9.8	754	9.8
Cardiopulmonary[b]	858	3.4	1 691	22.1
Dead on arrival	635	2.5	426	5.6
Other medical	10 626	42.3	2 933	38.3
Obstetric	173	0.7	23	0.3
Orthopedic	688	2.7	97	1.3
Injury	8 855	35.2	1 523	19.8
Refused aid	818	3.3	220	2.9
Total patients seen	25 113		7 667	
Patients transported	8 868	35	4 006	52
Assists	3 080		2 606	
No patients seen[c]	4 498		4 149	

[a] Seizures, CVAs, drug overdoses, psychiatric
[b] Suspected myocardial infarction, pulmonary edema, chronic lung disease
[c] False alarm, patient gone on arrival, run cancelled.

meeting' styled after the 'morning report' familiar to Medical House Officers. Analogous to that of an Intern, the men attend such sessions following the night 'on-call'. They hear didactic presentations and have an opportunity to present their cases of the previous night.

It might be noted that the last five to seven years have witnessed a steady evolution of emergency care in the surrounding Columbus suburbs. Most have developed their own Medic Units, and many have at least Squad units with EMT-A capability. Cooperation with units within the Columbus system has been established whereby more experienced men from the city units are able to supplement the training of those in the outlying areas.

Table 3. Columbus Medic Protocol for the management of patients with chest pain

I.   *Routine for all patients with suspected acute cardiopulmonary disease*
         1. Vital signs (BP, HR, Resp.)
         2. 12-lead ECG
         3. Start IV with D_5W (Dextrose water)
         4. O_2: 5–10 l/min (2 l/min for patients with lung disease)

II.   *Suspected myocardial infarction*
         1. If PVC's are a) frequent (>4/min)
                      b) multifocal
                      c) of a R on T pattern
                      d) 2 or more in a row
         then lidocaine (1 mg/kg) bolus is given for a 1 min period.
         After first bolus a lidocaine infusion (2 mg/cc IV fluid) should be given at a rate of 2 mg/min. After 10 min one-half of original bolus should be repeated.
         2. Bradycardia (<50/min)
           a) Sinus, nodal, $2°$ or $3°$ block – atropine 0.6–1.0 mg IV or IM should be given. If no response in 5 min, isoproterenol infusion (no more than 1 microgram/min) should be started.
           b) Atropine should be administered before lidocaine if patient with PVC's has bradycardia.

III.   *Suspected angina*
         1. Unstable angina
            – recent onset
            – first attack of angina
            – worsening of stable angina
            – spontaneous angina (onset at rest)
            – angina not responding to nitroglycerin (NTG)
              (after 2 tabs in 15 min.)
           a) Patient should always be transported by Medic (even with normal ECG) especially if he is a male over 35. If he refuses transportation, an effort should be made to contact a physician.
           b) Treatment
              1. Nitroglycerin 1/200 gr sublingually, which may be repeated 1 time, 5 to 10 min after initial dose.
              2. O_2:5–10l/min if pain persists.
         2. Chronic stable angina
           If patient responds promptly to nitroglycerin with no acute changes in the ECG, transportation should be offered.

Table 4. Acute myocardial infarction comparison of Heartmobile with Medic

	Heartmobile	Medic	P
No. of patients	191	83	NS
Age (in years)	63.5	63.5	NS
White men (%)	61	63	NS
Median decision time (min)	55	30	0.01
call to arrival (min)	12	6	0.01
Percentage seen by 2 hr	69	68	NS
Chest pain as chief complaint (%)	76	63	NS
Syncope as chief complaint (%)	6.5	21	<0.01
False-negative diagnosis of acute myocardial infarction (%)	13	17	NS
False-positive diagnosis of acute myocardial infarction (%)	58	44	<0.05
Patients with acute myocardial infarction and cardiac arrest (%)[a]	23	38	0.025
Overall mortality (%) (excluding emergency room deaths)	21.4	31.4	NS
Prehospital shock or cardiac arrest (%)	50	56.4	NS
Others (%)	11.8	15.6	NS
Patients with no serious complications (%)	70	54	0.02
Long-term survivors (%)			
Ventricular fibrillation	6	8.5	NS
Other cause of cardiac arrest	1	3.5	NS
Life-threatening events[b]	9	12.0	NS
Total	16	24.0	NS

[a] Includes patients who did not survive to admission.

[b] Includes all patients with coma due to circulatory collapse either at the time of or subsequent to the arrival of the emergency medical service. Excludes asystole unresponsive to therapy.

6. A COMPARISON OF PHYSICIANS AND AUTONOMOUS PARAMEDICS

The original Heartmobile® included a physician, and operation of this unit was compared with that subsequently obtained by autonomous Paramedics. A fifteen-month period (between October 1969 and December 1970) during which the Heartmobile® operated with a physician and three paramedics was compared with a three-month interval (March through May 1972) during which there were three Medic Vehicles each with three paramedics and no doctor [8]. Table 4 compares patients with acute myocardial infarction seen during these two periods of time. The reduced response time made possible during the 'medic period' is evident and significant (P = 0.01). The paramedics were as accurate as the doctor in diagnosing the exclusion of acute myocardial infarction. The paramedics were actually better in defining acute myocardial infarction. The overall mortality from myocardial infarction was higher during the Medic Unit operation, although not significantly so, and probably relates to the higher incidence of patients with serious complications seen by the Medic system. There was no difference in the percentage of patients who became long-term survivors of ventricular fibrillation and those who survived cardiac arrest and life-threatening events defined as patients with coma due to circulatory collapse when managed by either system.

Given an equal outcome relative to the care of patients with myocardial infarction, it also became very clear that the performance of manual skills was significantly better in the hands of well-trained paramedics [9].

In order to maintain the quality of care and paramedic skills, the previously described weekly medic meetings are supplemented by a review of all EMS runs by the Nurse Coordinator and the Battalion Chief of the EMS branch, and of selected runs by the Medical Director. Probably more important, however, is the frequent, repetitive, high volume exposure to similar types of emergencies, as well as the multi-tiered system which guarantees multiple personnel on the scene of any pre-hospital crisis. The role of the older paramedic with a decade of experience cannot be overestimated, and probably constitutes the most important element for the on-going success of the system.

7. A COMPARISON OF USERS AND NON-USERS OF COLUMBUS EMS

There remains little doubt that lives are saved by pre-hospital mobile coronary care units such as the one described in Columbus, Ohio [3–8, 10–14]. Many such systems have now proliferated in the United States and Europe [15, 16] but despite this, there remains uncertainty regarding the impact of pre-hospital care on mortality from myocardial infarction and sudden death in patients with coronary artery disease. It has even been suggested that such mobile units serve patients at low risk of dying who could be treated as easily by other means [17].

During the operation and evolution of the Columbus System [7–9], it was our impression that persons served by the Medic Units were predominantly those at very high risk of death. In order to address this problem as well as questions concerning cost efficacy and citizen abuse of the system, a prospective study was conducted during the years 1976 and 1977 [18]. This comprehensive, city-wide five hospital study was undertaken to review the course of patients with acute cardiac symptomatology and with the possible diagnosis of acute myocardial infarction. Case records of 1 102 patients were studied and two equal groups of 'users' and 'non-users' were matched for age, sex, and race. This sample represented only one fourth of the patients seen by the system in one year. Users were defined as patients who perceived a cardiac emergency sufficient to warrant their activation of the system described. Non-users were those patients who chose to present themselves to hospital by alternate means such as the family vehicle, private ambulance, or public transportation. This difference in the use and non-use of the system was found despite the fact that 96% of the non-users were aware of the system's availability.

Table 5. Percentage of acute coronary events seen by Columbus ALS Units (1976–1977)

	Estimated	Seen	% of total
	(no./yr)	(no./yr)	
AMI without prehospital sudden death	1438[a] (2.55/1000 pop.)	815[c]	57
CAD with prehospital sudden death	439[b] (0.78/1000 pop.)	257[d]	59
Overall	1877 (3.33/1000 pop.)	1072	57

ALS, Advanced Life Support
AMI, Acute Myocardial Infarction
CAD, Coronary Artery Disease

[a] Estimate obtained from Physician Activity Survey (PAS) data from all Columbus hospitals.
[b] Based upon a 1970 epidemiologic study of sudden death in Columbus including only those with symptoms less than 1–2 h.
[c] Estimated from annual Fire Department statistics.
[d] Estimated from annual Fire Department statistics including only patients in whom resuscitation was possible.

Records of all patients were carefully reviewed by a nurse epidemiologist. All electrocardiograms were collected, and all patients or families were interviewed during the hospital course as well as six months later. The records of all patients were then analyzed by two independent physician reviewers so as to determine the ultimate diagnosis. Thus a group of 544 patients was generated who had suffered acute myocardial infarction and who became the focus of the study. Diagnosis of myocardial infarction was dependent upon typical symptomatology, electrocardiographic change, and serum enzyme determinations. If no Q-waves developed despite appropriate enzyme elevation, the patient was considered to have had a non-transmural infarction. When left bundle branch block or other QRS deformities preventing precise electrocardiographic diagnosis were present, the patient was considered to have sustained infarction provided that a compatible history and enzyme patterns were found.

Table 5 illustrates an estimate of the expected number of acute coronary events in the population of Columbus obtained from hospital discharge statistics during the period of the 1976–77 study, and from a study of sudden deaths in the Columbus community [19]. A review of Fire Department records indicates that the Medic Units see approximately 57% of infarction patients who do not experience sudden death and 59% of coronary sudden death cases. This contrasts with the experience gained with the original 1970 Heartmobile® when only 10% of each category of patients was seen.

Table 6 illustrates the difference between users and non-users. Noteworthy is the time difference from onset of symptomatology to initiation of definitive care (arrival

110

Table 6. Distribution of selected characteristics of patients admitted to the hospital with AMI (1976–1977)

	Users	Non-users
N	274	270
Age	62.6±12	61.3±11
Male percentage	69	77[b]
Time Onset Sx to Rx	45 min	252 min[b]
Percentage with incapacitating Sx	55	37[b]
Percentage with transmural MI	71	71
Percentage with peak SGOT >100	55	33[b]
Percentage with serious complications[a]	53	16[b]
Hospital mortality (excluding emergency room deaths)	16.7%	1.5%[b]

Rx, Arrival of MCCU or arrival at hospital emergency room for non-users.
Sx, symptoms.

[a] Cardiac arrest, pulmonary edema, shock, hypotension-bradycardia syndrome (includes pre-hospital and new hospital events).
[b] Significant at $p < 0.05$ (users vs. non-users).

of the medic for the users or arrival of non-users at the hospital emergency room). Although the presenting symptoms were similar for both groups, the users more frequently had symptoms judged 'incapacitating'; this of course was part of the reason for summoning the Medic Units in the first place. The incidence of transmural myocardial infarction was the same in the two groups, while the number of patients with striking enzyme rises and serious complications was significantly greater in the user group. These indicators of patients being 'more ill' when seen by the EMS system is borne out by the striking difference between users and non-users with respect to hospital mortality. The unprecedented low hospital mortality for the non-user group of 1.5% indicates the benignity of the illness in these patients and, perhaps, their appropriate election not to activate the EMS system. This is a delicate point, but probably it is an intriguing result of public education simply pointing to prudent and optimized usage of a pre-hospital mobile coronary care system by those patients most ill and most in need of complex care.

8. THE IMPACT OF PRUDENT PATIENT ACTIVATION ON THE COMMUNITY MORTALITY OF MYOCARDIAL INFARCTION

The determination of the impact of mobile coronary care on the mortality from myocardial infarction has been one of the most difficult questions to answer [12, 20]. Some have gone so far as to suggest that taking patients to the hospital is no better than treating patients with myocardial infarction in the home [21]. There are very

Table 7. Types of acute myocardial infarction among users and non-users

MI Type	Users		Non-users	
	N	Total (%)	N	Total (%)
Anterolateral transmural	81	29.5	95	35.0
Inferoposterior transmural	115	42.0	97	36.0
LBBB and other[a]	38	14.0	31	11.5
Non-transmural	40	14.5	47	17.5
Total	274	100	270	100

[a] Infarct could not be localized due to prior infarction(s).

important questions that relate to the data presented in the study by Adgey [22] and our results would suggest that a different result occurs from use of a combined system of pre-hospital and hospital coronary care.

The distribution of the types of myocardial infarction reported in the most recent study sample is shown in Table 7, there being no significant differences between users and non-users. Table 8 illustrates the incidence of major complications and case fatality rates associated with these complications in the user and non-user groups. Many patients had more than one major complication, and an attempt was made therefore to assign only the complication which was the primary cause of

Table 8. Site, incidence, and case fatality rate of complications among users and non-users[a]

	Users						Non-users			Total		
	Pre-hospital			Hospital			Hospital			Users and non-users		
	N	Compli. % of total users	CFR (%)	N	Compli. % of total users[a]	CFR (%)	N	Compli. % of total non-users	CFR (%)	N	Compli. % of total users and non-users	CFR (%)
VF or CA	38	14	45	26	9.5	62	20	7.4	10	84	15.4	41.5
Cardiogenic shock	9	3.3	33	7	2.6	71	5	1.9	40	21	3.9	47.5
Hypo-brady	28	10.2	7	10	3.3	0	13	4.8	0	51	9.4	3.9
Pulmonary edema	17	6.2	18	11	4.0	0	4	1.5	0	32	5.9	9.5
Total	92	33.7		54	19.4		42	15.6		188	34.6	

Compli, Complication
CFR, Case fatality rate (%) (excluding emergency room deaths)
VF, Ventricular fibrillation
CA, Cardiac arrest not due to VF
Hypo-brady, Hypotension-bradycardia syndrome

[a] Only new complications developing after hospitalization are listed.

Table 9. The impact of EMS on mortality of acute myocardial infarction (AMI)

Fatalities among 156 AMI patients	46 users (includes 17 (45%) of 38 with pre-hospital arrest)
	4 non-users
	30 died in ER (and did not survive to permit admission and substantiation of the diagnosis of AMI)
	47 died suddenly and were not seen (41% of sudden death victims)[a]
	29 died at home, not suddenly (3.6% of total AMI)[b]
Total of 804 patients	544 study group
(30 + 47)	77 sudden death
(19.2% of total AMI)[b]	154 non-fatal AMI at home and not seen
(3.6% of total AMI)[b]	29 died at home, not suddenly

The proportion of 156 to 804 is 19% of the overall one-year city-wide mortality of AMI patients.

[a] If 59% of patients with sudden death were seen (see Table 5), then $0.59 X = 68$ (i.e. 30 + 38) and $X = 115$; 47 patients (41%) were not seen.
[b] Based on Framingham experience.

death. Users experienced a 34% pre-hospital rate of serious complications, and an additional 19% experienced 'new complications' following hospital admission. Comparison with the non-user group reiterates that the user group was 'more ill'. In the total cohort of users and non-users serious complications occurred in only 34.6%, and the incidence of cardiogenic shock was very low at 4%. This is to be contrasted with numbers obtained in patient populations that are more selected than in this community-wide study.

There were 68 initially successful pre-hospital resuscitations of patients with coronary artery disease in the study sample. Ninety-two percent had ventricular fibrillation. Thirty patients died before admission to the hospital and another 17 died after admission. Twenty-one patients (31%) were discharged from the hospital alive, and the six-month case fatality rate for the survivors of pre-hospital ventricular fibrillation who were discharged alive was 19%.

It is difficult to estimate the impact of the Columbus EMS system on overall community mortality from ischemic heart disease. Reliable data on expected mortality in the 1970's are not available. The striking decline in mortality since 1970 [23] renders earlier epidemiologic studies less useful [24]. If the Framingham experience is used in terms of 100 patients with myocardial infarction, a comparison figure for overall city-wide mortality of first myocardial infarction of 30.5% is obtained. This figure would include 39 patients not hospitalized, among whom 19.2 with non-fatal events and 3.6 who die at home though not suddenly. Of the 61 hospitalized, 11% die. Extrapolation of these figures to the 1976–77 study in Columbus, Ohio, yields estimated data as shown in Table 9. This estimation includes the Framingham guidelines as well as the estimated 59% of total patients with pre-hospital sudden death seen during the 1976–77 Columbus experience. The total population with acute myocardial infarction with regard to these estimates was based upon our study sample of users and non-users which represented only one fourth of the actual patients with infarction in one year. Using these guidelines, the overall oneyear citywide mortality from acute myocardial infarction approximates 19%, which compares quite favorably with figures as high as 50% in the past.

Crampton has emphasized the difficulty of estimating the number of lives saved by prompt treatment of complications other than cardiac arrest [20]. If only the patients in Columbus with pre-hospital cardiac arrest are considered, 21 of 68 of patients (31%) in whom initial resuscitation was successful were discharged alive (7.66% of the user group). With reference to Table 5 and the fact that a total of 257 patients with pre-hospital arrest due to coronary artery disease were seen during the year of the study, the 31% save rate may be extrapolated to 80 lives saved overall for the year[1]. Based on a population of $564\,871$[2] this corresponds to 14.2 lives saved from coronary sudden death per $100\,000$ population per year. By six months, 4 of 21 survivors had died reducing the figures to 25% save rate and 11.4 per $100\,000$ per year. The cost to achieve this result is below $ 1 000 per life saved. This apparently favorable result may not be realized when only a small proportion of myocardial infarction patients are seen [25] or when patient delay obviates the benefits of pre-hospital care in the earliest hours of infarction [26].

9. OUT-OF-HOSPITAL ELECTROCARDIOGRAMS AND BRETYLIUM TOSYLATE IN REFRACTORY VENTRICULAR FIBRILLATION

9.1. The pre-hospital intermediate syndrome

One of the unmistakable features of the Columbus mobile coronary care experience has been the observation of striking electrocardiograms in the pre-hospital setting, with tracings not being reproduced in the subsequent course of the patient. These electrocardiograms sometimes become the most important objective criteria of ischemic heart disease in a given patient, and are gained by the paramedics seeing patients during the most acute phase of their illness (Figure 5). Table 10 illustrates the utility of the pre-hospital electrocardiogram as obtained in the aforementioned user study. It is seen that only 12% of patients with acute myocardial infarction had a normal pre-hospital electrocardiogram, and 8% of patients with transmural infarction.

---

[1] Not all patients with myocardial infarction during the year could be identified and included in the final study group of 274 patients. The total figures in Tables 5 and 9 should not be expected to correspond exactly.

[2] 1980 Census Bureau published figure for City of Columbus proper.

114

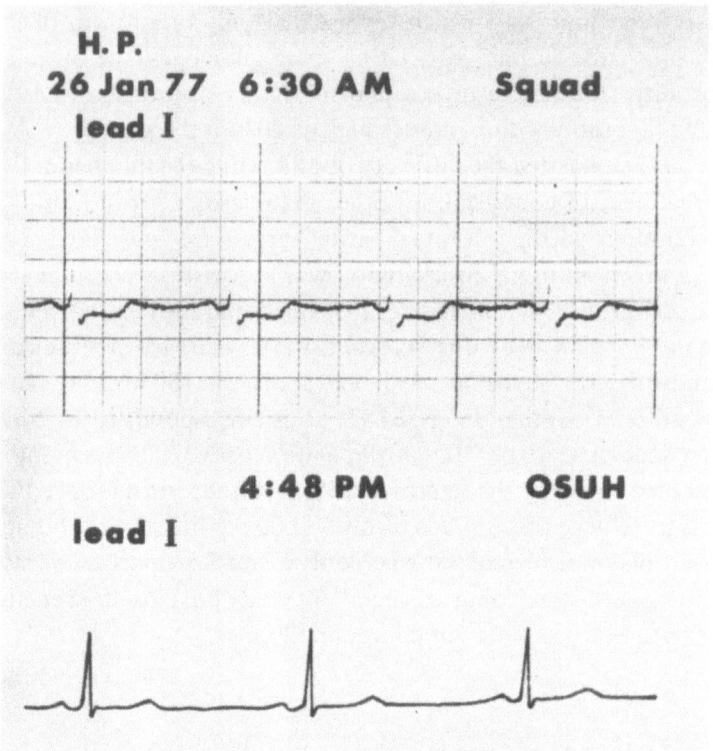

Figure 5. A comparison of pre-hospital and hospital electrocardiograms (ECG) in the same patient. The ST-segment depression seen in the former tracings was the sole spontaneous ECG change recorded in this patient.

9.2. *The use of 'monitor' quality vs. 'diagnostic quality' electrocardiograms*

One possible criticism of the paramedic pre-hospital use of electrocardiograms as a diagnostic tool might relate to their use of equipment capable only of so called 'monitor quality'. In anticipation of this, a study recently has been conducted employing not only the customary portable equipment (Lifepak® − 5; Physio-Control, Redmond, Wash.) but also a device (Lifepak® − 6) permitting sequential (and therefore nearly simultaneous) tracings of both types (delay and real time) as follows:

Lifepak® − 6	Type of tracing	Frequency response
Monitor quality	Delay	0.5–40 Hz
Diagnostic quality	Real Time	0.05–100 Hz

Six patients were seen where all three tracings could safely be obtained. In all six, no important differences in QRS morphology, ST-segment deviation, or T-wave change were seen. An example of one such patient is shown in Figure 6.

Although we have not been able to document accurately, we have been told that the customary portable 'monitor quality' electrocardiographic equipment will sometimes exaggerate ST-segment shifts, seemingly artifactually. If true, this could partially explain the apparent high frequency of 'abnormal' pre-hospital tracings previously mentioned. At worst, this would prompt the paramedics to err unwittingly and conservatively on the side of too cautious overdiagnosis. There are certainly no data to support the reverse phenomenon.

9.3. The use of bretylium tosylate in the pre-hospital therapy of refractory ventricular fibrillation

In the spring of 1981, the Advisory Council approved of a modification to the protocol for the treatment of refractory ventricular fibrillation (VF). Patients remaining in refractory VF have since been treated with 5 mg/kg of bretylium tosylate given as an intravenous bolus which was repeated when necessary in 10 min. When necessary defibrillation is attempted again. In our early experience we were confronted with eleven such patients six of whom were converted to an effective rhythm and thereby not transported in VF. Obviously, our initial impressions have been favorable. The paper by Cobb and his colleagues subsequent to these experiences has shown in great detail a close comparability of bretylium with lidocaine as a firstline drug [27]. Our experience has shown the role of this drug in the effective treatment of patients who are otherwise brought to the hospital in case of persistent VF. Others have reported so-called 'pharmacologic defibrillations' after bretylium [28]. This was observed in one of our patients.

Table 10. The utility of the pre-hospital electrocardiogram (ECG)[a]

	ST ↑	ST ↓	Normal ECG
Anterior transmural	34/55 (62%)	14/55 (25%)	7/55 (13%)
Inferior transmural	72/93 (77%)	16/93 (17%)	5/93 (5%)
Non-transmural	8/27 (30%)	10/27 (37%)	9/27 (33%)
Total			21/175
Incidence of normal pre-hospital ECG:			12%
Incidence of normal pre-hospital ECG (in transmural AMI):			8%

[a] Analysis restricted to those with an adequate and complete pre-hospital tracing; patients with left bundle branch block, paced rhythm, etc. were excluded.

116

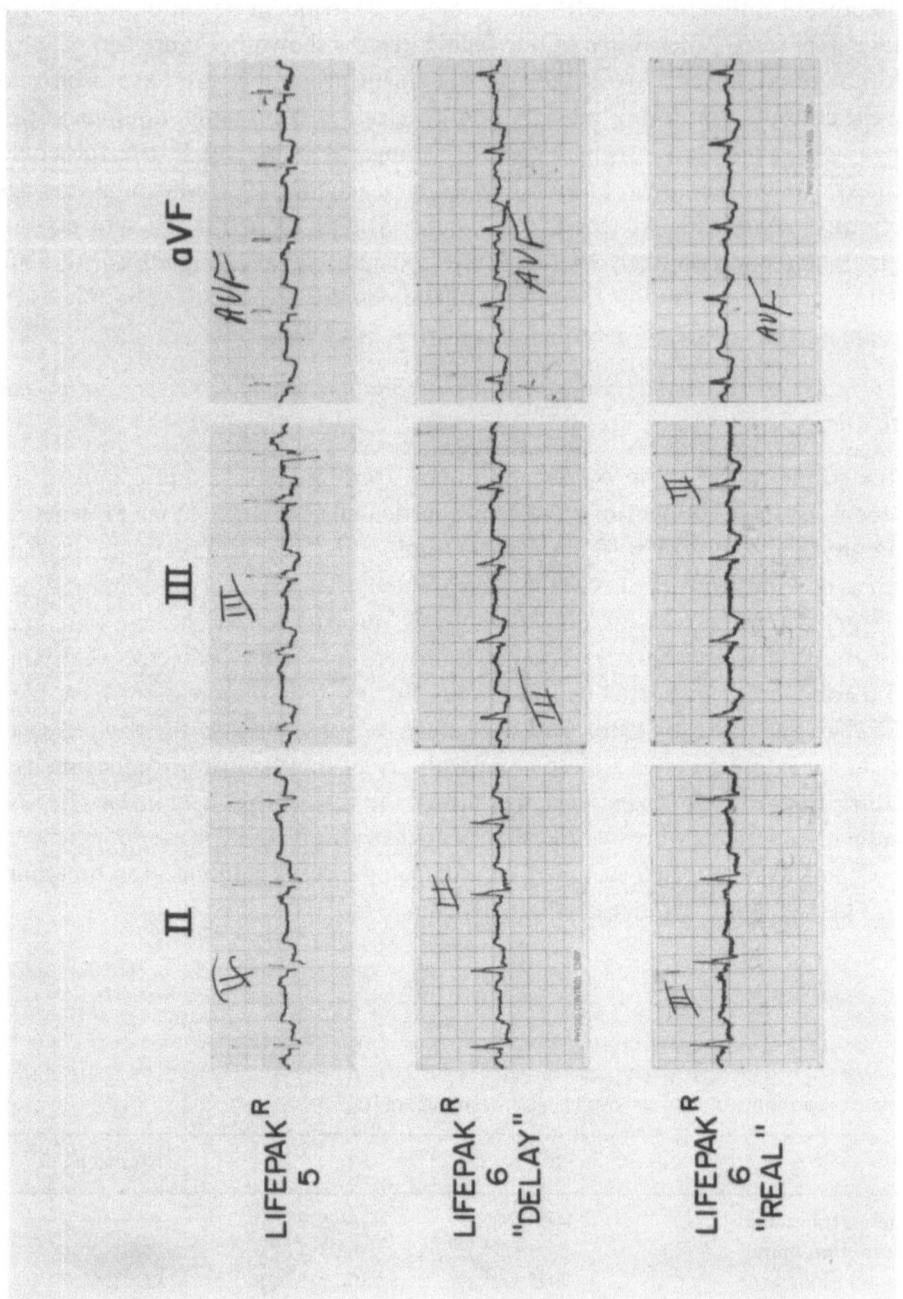

Figure 6. A comparison of near-simultaneous, pre-hospital ECG tracings in leads II, III, and aVF in a single patient with chest pain and possible myocardial infarction. No important difference is seen in the 1–2 mm ST segment depression, T wave inversion, and intraventricular conduction defect between the three different techniques.

10. SUMMARY AND FUTURE DIRECTIONS

More than a decade of pre-hospital coronary care in this city as well as in others has yielded an extraordinary amount of experience in a totally new field of medical care. So called 'survivors of sudden death' are now commonplace, and the overall mortality of ischemic heart disease is indeed falling [23], at least partly, by virtue of these efforts. This pre-hospital care can be delivered by paramedics working independently of the immediate presence of a physician. The community mortality of myocardial infarction may be reduced. Efforts to reach all potential victims are perhaps tempered by the observation that, with the exception of victims of sudden death not seen, voluntary 'non-users' may be patients who by public education in a 'saturated' community have correctly perceived the benignity of their illness. Future goals should be pursued with the following points in mind:
1. Improved public education in basic life support concepts and techniques.
2. Improved EMS programs for rural areas.
3. Freer access by laymen to resuscitative devices, perhaps including defibrillatory equipment.
4. Continued efforts toward preventive therapy via risk factor identification and modification.
5. Fuller development of guidelines for the therapy of uncomplicated myocardial infarction seen within the first hour or hours from onset of symptoms.

Response to the urge for 'medical control' should be in terms of continued physician-directed monitoring and supervision of paramedics whose education is also directed by committed physicians. Telemetry, voice contact and pre-hospital presence of a physician should not be mandated but used rather selectively, commensurate with the characteristics of the community served.

ACKNOWLEDGEMENTS

The authors recognize the pioneering efforts of Dr. James V. Warren, M.D., who was uniquely responsible for the Heartmobile® and Columbus Mobile Coronary Care. Also recognized are the efforts of Battalion Chief Harmon J. Dutko, Kathryn L. Sampson, BSN, and Phillip K. Fulkerson, M.D. Special thanks are extended to Ms. Sharon Williams for manuscript preparation.

REFERENCES

1. Dodosh MN: Hello, Columbus. Thriving Ohio capital seeks to shed its image as a country bumkin. The Wall Street Journal 61 (34):1 and 19, 1980.
2. Day HW: An intensive coronary care area. Dis Chest 44:423–427, 1963.
3. Pantridge JF, Geddes JS: Cardiac arrest after myocardial infarction. Lancet 1:807–808, 1966.

118

4. Pantridge JF, Geddes JS: A mobile intensive-care unit in the management of myocardial infarction. Lancet 2:271–273, 1967.
5. Grace WJ: The mobile coronary care unit and the intermediate coronary care unit in the total systems approach to coronary care. Chest 58:363–368, 1970.
6. McMullen JB, Lewis RP, Mattingly CV, Warren JV: Experience with a mobile coronary care unit. Ann Intern Med 72:779–780, 1970. (Abstract.)
7. Lewis RP, Fulkerson PK, Stang JM, Sampson KL, Dutko HJ: The Columbus emergency medical service system. Ohio State Med J 75:391–394, 1979.
8. Lewis RP, Stang JM, Fulkerson PK, Sampson KL, Scoles A, Warren JV: Effectiveness of advanced paramedics in a mobile coronary care system. JAMA 241:1902–1904, 1979.
9. DeLeo BC: Endotracheal intubation by rescue squad personnel. Heart Lung 6:851–854, 1977.
10. Liberthson RR, Nagel EL, Hirschman JC, Nussenfeld SR: Prehospital ventricular defibrillation. Prognosis and follow-up course. N Engl J Med 291:317–321, 1974.
11. Baum RS, Alvarez H III, Cobb LA: Survival after resuscitation from out-of-hospital ventricular fibrillation. Circulation 50:1231–1235, 1974.
12. Crampton RS, Aldrich RF, Gascho JA, Miles JR Jr, Stillerman R: Reduction of prehospital, ambulance and community coronary death rates by the community-wide emergency cardiac care system. Am J Med 58:151–165, 1975.
13. Mackintosh AF, Crabb ME, Grainger R, Williams JH, Chamberlain DA: The Brighton resuscitation ambulances: review of 40 consecutive survivors of out-of-hospital cardiac arrest. Br Med J 1:1115–1118, 1978.
14. McNeill GP, Boucher IAD, Watson H: Mobile coronary care available to the general public. Lancet 1:975, 1979.
15. Pantridge JF, Adgey AAJ, Geddes JS, Webb SW: The Acute Coronary Attack. pp. 130–131. Tunbridge Wells: Pitman Medical, 1975.
16. Hoffer EP: Emergency Medical Services, 1979. N Engl J Med 301:1118–1121, 1979.
17. Hampton JR, Dowling M, Nicholas C: Comparison of results from a cardiac ambulance manned by medical or non-medical personnel. Lancet 1:526–529, 1977.
18. Lewis RP, Stang JM, Keller MD, Lanese RR, Chirikos TN, Warren JV: Reduction of mortality from myocardial infarction by prudent patient activation of mobile coronary care. Am Heart J 103:123–130, 1982.
19. Keller MD, Bashe W: Sudden cardiac death and onset of myocardial infarction. A clinical pathological correlation. Myocardial Infarction Branch, National Heart and Lung Institute, February 1972.
20. Crampton R: Prehospital advanced cardiac life support: evaluation of a decade of experience. Topics in Emergency Medicine 1:27–36, 1980.
21. Hill JD, Hampton JR, Mitchell JRA: A randomized trial of home vs. hospital management of patients with suspected myocardial infarction. Lancet 1:837–841, 1978.
22. Adgey AAJ: Effective coronary care and mortality rates. Am Heart J 100:408, 1980.
23. Stern MP: The recent decline in ischemic heart disease mortality. Ann Intern Med 91:630–640, 1979.
24. Kannel WB, Castelli WP, McNamara PM: Epidemiology of acute myocardial infarction. Medicine Today 2:56–70, 1968.
25. Vetter NH, Pocock S, Julian DG: Measuring the effect of a mobile coronary care unit upon the community. Br Heart J 41:418–25, 1979.
26. Siltanen P, Sundberg S, Hytönen I: Impact of a mobile coronary care unit on the sudden coronary mortality in a community. Acta Med Scand 205:195–200, 1979.
27. Haynes RE, Chinn TL, Copass MK, Cobb LA: Comparison of bretylium tosylate and lidocaine in management of out of hospital ventricular fibrillation: A randomized clinical trial. Am J Cardiol 48:353–356, 1981.
28. Holder DA, Sniderman AD, Fraser G, Fallen EL: Experience with bretylium tosylate by a hospital cardiac arrest team. Circulation 55:541–544, 1977.

7. PREHOSPITAL CORONARY CARE IN THE VIRGINIA PIEDMONT AND UNITED STATES

RICHARD S. CRAMPTON

1. INTRODUCTION

During the 16 years since the inception of prehospital coronary care in Belfast, Northern Ireland [1, 2], the lives of thousands of acutely ill cardiac patients have been saved and their quality of life has been improved by a lowered morbidity. Nowhere has this been more apparent than in the United States where Pantridge's concept of mobile coronary care revolutionized emergency medical services. The ease of detection of prefatal and fatal arrhythmias in acute ischemic heart disease and the portability of the relevant instruments and drugs to monitor, defibrillate and treat the coronary patient, expedited experimental emergency care systems staffed first by physicians and then by nurses, paramedics and emergency medical technicians (EMTs). Since costs, benefits and outcomes were easily assessed, innovative improvements attended rapid feedback of favorable results. This chapter will discuss the adaptation of mobile coronary care in the Virginia Piedmont, the United States, Canada and Europe, the influence of cardiopulmonary resuscitation (CPR) by the citizen, the noncontroversy about mobile coronary care, the financial burden and benefit to the community, and the important role of the physician who is responsible for medical control of prehospital coronary care.

2. PREHOSPITAL CORONARY CARE IN THE VIRGINIA PIEDMONT

In March 1971, volunteer rescue workers serving the city of Charlottesville and the county of Albemarle and resident physicians of the University Hospital began Virginia's first systematic, comprehensive, community wide, prehospital coronary care system. The community of 80 000 people comprised a city of 40 000 inhabitants with suburban and rural districts in the county. The area served was 745 square miles (2068 km²). The rescue workers provided transport and basic life support (CPR) and physicians and nurses provided advanced cardiac life support. We modelled our prehospital system for emergency cardiac care (ECC) upon the mobile coronary care unit (MCCU) initiated in 1966 at the Royal Victoria Hospital, Belfast, Northern Ireland [1, 2], added it to our extant ambulance service [3–8], and modified it drawing upon the experiences in experimental medical, paramedical and basic emergency services in Miami, Seattle, Columbus, New York, Los Angeles and Virginia Beach [9–18].

Adgey, AAJ (ed): Acute phase of ischemic heart disease and myocardial infarction.
© 1982, Martinus Nijhoff, The Hague, Boston, London. ISBN-13: 978-94-009-7581-1

2.1. Results in the Virginia Piedmont

Table 1 records deaths from 1960 to 1974 due to ischemic heart disease in the Commonwealth of Virginia and in the Charlottesville-Albemarle community from figures compiled by Doctor John Alexander, Public Health Resident, Thomas Jefferson Health District. In 1966 hospital coronary care began in the Charlottesville-Albemarle community, but predictably did not reduce the community mortality from coronary disease [19, 20]. Subsequently, we developed the rationale for mobile coronary care in our community from two sources. First, data collected during the first three years of service of the MCCU at the Royal Victoria Hospital, Belfast documented a reduction in coronary mortality [21]. Secondly, since coronary deaths before and after the introduction of hospital coronary units did not alter the overall coronary mortality in the community (Table 1, Figure 1) [19, 20], we calculated, using Pantridge's estimate [21], the theoretical reduction in the frequency of out-of-hospital and inhospital coronary death by provision of MCCU service to our community (Figure 2) [22]. We predicted a 27% reduction in community mortality if the frequency of prehospital deaths during the first two hours after onset of symptoms was diminished. In our survey, preventable deaths at the patient-ambulance interface and in the emergency room contributed to the potential reduction of coronary mortality by the MCCU (Figure 2).

Table 1. Deaths from ischemic heart disease, 1960–1974

Commonwealth of Virginia			City of Charlottesville and Albemarle County				
Year	Deaths N	Population	Death rate per 100 000	Deaths N	Population	Death rate per 100 000	Expected deaths N	Expected death rate per 100 000
1960	9,925	3,983,160	249	172	60,396	285	169	280
1961	9,953	4,036,326	247	177	62,022	285	180	290
1962	10,667	4,126,150	259	214	63,648	336	193	303
1963	11,149	4,237,473	263	210	65,274	322	202	309
1964	11,192	4,307,591	260	243	66,900	363	204	305
1965	11,323	4,425,637	256	186	68,526	271	207	302
Hospital coronary care introduced in 1966								
1966	11,838	4,525,976	262	216	70,152	308	194	277
1967	11,985	4,602,091	260	195	71,778	272	198	276
1968	12,557	4,692,675	268	220	73,404	300	208	283
1969	13,003	4,781,175	272	202	75,030	269	217	289
1970	13,169	4,665,532	282	225	76,660	294	232	303
Prehospital basic and advanced life support began in 1971								
1971	13,252	4,714,227	281	192	78,722	244	235	299
1972	13,403	4,764,000	281	199	80,840	246	242	299
1973	13,502	4,811,000	281	188	83,014	226	258	311
1974	13,281	4,908,000	271	217	85,247	255	245	287

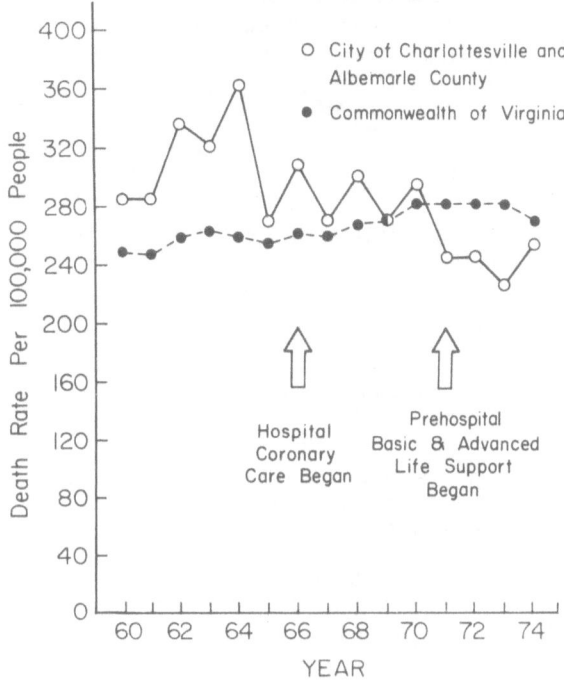

Figure 1. Yearly coronary deaths did not fall significantly after introduction of hospital coronary care units in the Charlottesville-Albemarle community in 1966. Upon addition of prehospital basic and advanced life support in 1971, coronary deaths (white dots) declined in the Charlottesville-Albemarle community in contrast to Virginia (black dots).

In 1971 prehospital basic and advanced life support began in our community as part of its extant emergency medical service. Figure 1 indicates that upon introduction of the MCCU, coronary death rate for Charlottesville-Albemarle fell while coronary death rate for Virginia remained the same. Figure 3 illustrates the decline in observed coronary death rate when compared with expected deaths for Charlottesville-Albemarle after the commencement of prehospital coronary care. Figure 4 indicates the fall in ambulance deaths from coronary disease after initiation of prehospital basic and advanced life support. For 1971 and 1972, the significant decrease of coronary deaths at the patient-ambulance interface occurred when compared with the assumed fatal outcome in the absence of the MCCU. It is remarkable that in 1973 the reduction in coronary deaths was significant whether or not resuscitation at the patient-ambulance interface was counted (Figure 4). Either coronary death declined spontaneously as suggested by a national trend or very early emergency cardiac care precluded the development of cardiopulmonary arrest due to ventricular fibrillation or asystole as predicted [21] and as confirmed by careful cumulative observations [23]. That the decrease of coronary mortality cannot be attributed solely to a national trend is suggested by Figure 5. While coronary death rate rose in Virginia by 6%, it fell in Charlottesville and Albemarle County.

122

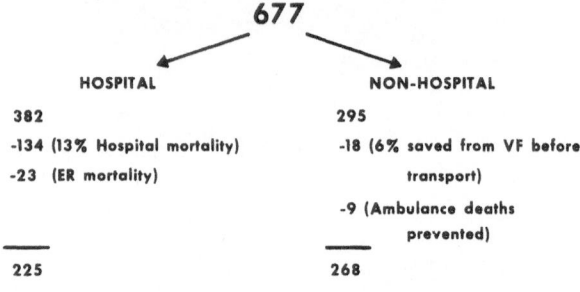

**THEORETICAL EFFECT OF MCCU
ON 1967 - 1969 CORONARY DEATHS**
Charlottesville & Albemarle County, Virginia

677

HOSPITAL   NON-HOSPITAL

382   295

-134 (13% Hospital mortality)   -18 (6% saved from VF before

-23   (ER mortality)   transport)

                         -9 (Ambulance deaths

                            prevented)

225   268

ADJUSTED CORONARY DEATHS

493

184 DEATHS PREVENTED
0.8 DEATHS/1000 POPULATION PREVENTED YEARLY
27% REDUCTION OF MORTALITY

Figure 2. From Pantridge's observations and predictions (21) and from our community-wide survey of preventable coronary deaths in the first 2 h of symptoms, the mobile coronary care unit (MCCU) theoretically would reduce community mortality from coronary disease by 27%. The frequency of fatal ventricular fibrillation (VF) would decline in non-hospital, emergency room (ER) and hospital phases of the coronary attack.

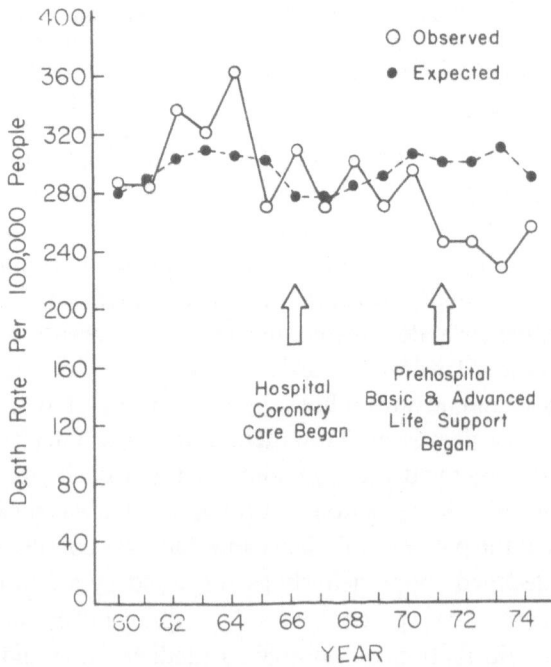

Figure 3. Upon introduction of prehospital basic and advanced life support to the Charlottesville-Albemarle community in 1971, yearly observed (white dots) coronary deaths fell significantly below expected (black dots) levels. In contrast, hospital coronary care alone (1966–70) made no difference.

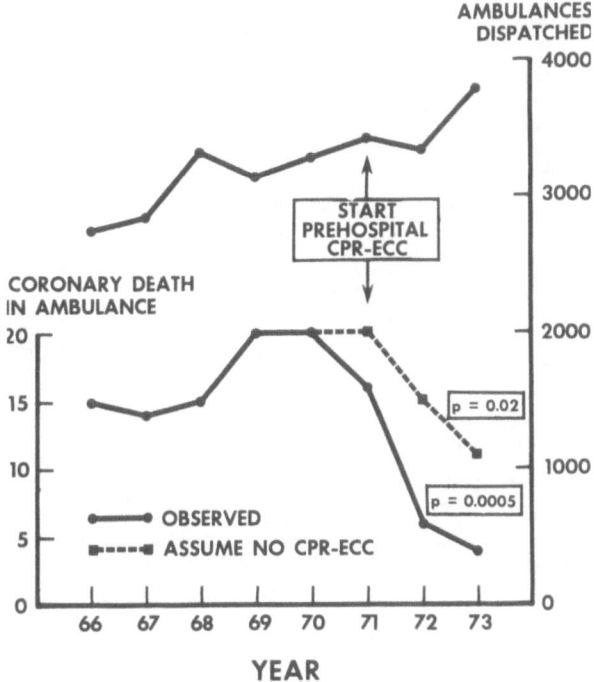

Figure 4. Yearly observed coronary deaths at the ambulance interface in people aged 30–69 years (lower solid line) are related to yearly number of ambulances dispatched from 1966 to 1973 (upper solid line). The significant fall (X^2, $p = 0.0005$) in coronary deaths in 1971–72 resulted from long-term (hospital) survivors of prehospital cardiopulmonary resuscitation (CPR) and emergency cardiac care (ECC). In 1973 the significant fall in coronary deaths irrespective of resuscitation (dashed line, $p = 0.02$) may reflect either a spontaneous decline in coronary death, or early prehospital drug therapy which averted cardiac arrest, or both.

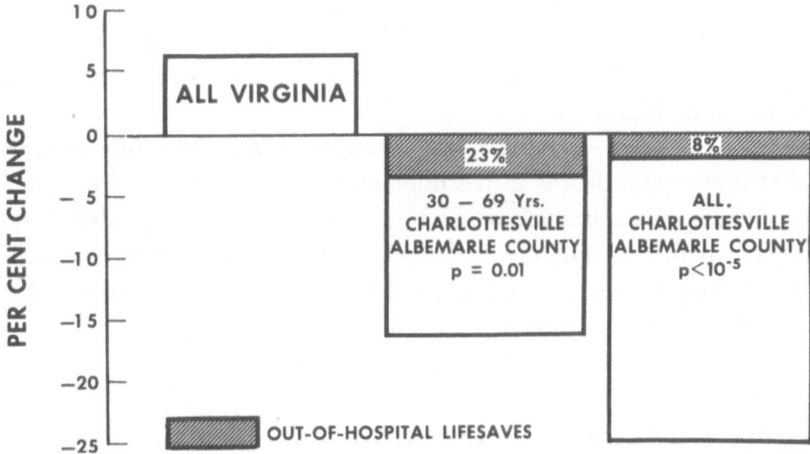

Figure 5. Out-of-hospital life saves by the MCCU from 1971 to 1973 contributed to the difference between the 6% rise (when compared with the years 1966–1970) in coronary deaths for Virginia (all ages) and the 16% (age 30–69 years) and 25% (all ages) fall in coronary deaths in Charlottesville and Albemarle County. (X^2 test of raw data).

124

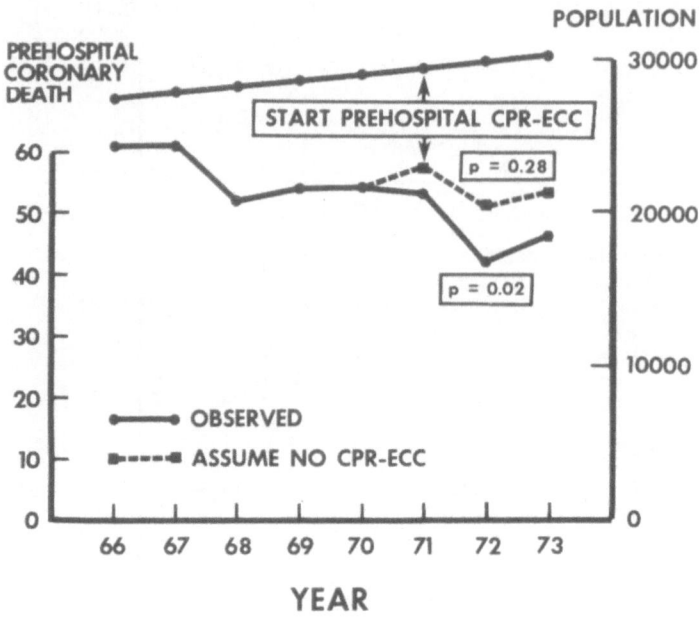

Figure 6. Yearly observed prehospital coronary deaths (lower solid line) from 1966 to 1973 in population aged 30–69 years (upper solid line). Prehospital cardiopulmonary resuscitation (CPR) and emergency cardiac care (ECC), introduced in 1971, significantly reduced out-of-hospital coronary deaths (X^2, $p = 0.02$). Absence of CPR-ECC confers death (dashed line, $p = 0.28$).

The fall in coronary deaths appeared most striking in the total population where prehospital resuscitation could account for only 8% of the long-term life saves. However, after isolation of nongeriatric coronary deaths (no coronary deaths occurred in people under 30 years of age), nearly one quarter of the reduction in coronary deaths in people aged 30–69 years was generated by the MCCU in out-of-hospital life saves (Figure 5).

Apparently initiation of prehospital coronary care significantly reduced the number of prehospital deaths in the population aged 30–69 years (Figure 6). If the identifiable prehospital life saves by the MCCU which yielded long-term (hospital) survivors were counted as number of prehospital deaths, no significant change would have occurred in the prehospital coronary death rate for the 30–69 age group (Figure 6).

3. PREHOSPITAL CORONARY CARE IN THE USA AND PREHOSPITAL CPR

When data from the USA are examined with respect to the level of training of the provider of ECC (Table 2), one cannot escape the impression that quantifiably positive results attend aggressive conduct of prehospital ECC at the community level. Although active in feasibility trials, physicians and nurses no longer provide prehospital ECC in most American communities. Paramedics, intermediate EMTs, and basic EMTs have been compared and the latter category of personnel are less effective than the former two categories [28, 30] (Table 2). When 10 h of training in the recognition of ventricular fibrillation and the delivery of transthoracic DC shocks were added to the basic 80 h EMT course, the number of long-term survivors significantly increased [28, 30]. However, conventional therapy in the prevention of cardiac arrest from ventricular fibrillation and asystole such as correcting acute dysautonomia, relieving ischemic chest pain and stabilizing rhythm should not be abandoned [5–8, 21, 23], since this practice by physicians and by certain paramedic systems has achieved superior results (Table 2).

Prehospital CPR substantially increases the number of long-term survivors of out-of-hospital cardiac arrest (Table 3) and also reduced morbidity [24]. For maximum benefit, basic life support (CPR) must be provided within 4 min of collapse from ventricular fibrillation and transthoracic DC shock delivered within 8 min of collapse [34] CPR is emphatically not an alternative to advanced life support. Both the Winnipeg and King County surveys conducted before addition of systematic advanced life support to each community indicate that only two to three life saves per 100 000 can be achieved by CPR alone with transport to the emergency department for defibrillation (Table 3). A good prehospital coronary care service should

Table 2. Influence of prehospital coronary care upon the community in the United States

Community	Yearly saves of life per 100 000 population	Ambulance personnel
Seattle, Washington	20.6[a]	Paramedic [24]
Columbus	14.2	Paramedic, EMT [25]
	5.0	Paramedic, EMT [26]
San Antonio	11.5	Paramedic [27]
King County	10.2 – 13.9	Paramedic, EMT [28]
Washington	12.3	Paramedic [29]
	7.2	EMT - defibrillator technician [30]
	2.6[b]	EMT [28, 30]
Charlottesville & Albemarle County, Virginia	6.8 & 14.8[c]	Physician, EMT [8]
Miami	6.3	Paramedic, EMT [31]
Los Angeles	5.2	Paramedic [27]
Cincinnati	4.9	Paramedic [27]
Minneapolis	4.4	Paramedic, EMT [32]

EMT = Emergency medical technician

[a] Includes ventricular fibrillation after arrival of paramedics.

[b] Basic life support only.

[c] 14.8 life-saves of persons aged 30–69 years per 100 000 people of this age group.

Table 3. Survival rates with and without prehospital cardiopulmonary resuscitation (CPR) by a citizen

Community	Cases (N)	Cardiac event	Discharge from Hospital	
			Citizen CPR	No citizen CPR
Oslo [33]	631	Unstated	27/75 (36%)	43/556 (8%)
Suburban Seattle [34]	487	All cardiac arrests	25/108 (23%)	45/379 (12%)
Seattle [24]	316	Ventricular fibrillation	47/109 (43%)	43/207 (21%)
Los Angeles [35]	120	Ventricular fibrillation	12/49 (24%)	4/71 (6%)
	170	Not documented as ventricular fibrillation	9/55 (16%)	3/115 (3%)
Winnipeg[a] [36]	226	Ventricular tachycardia and fibrillation	16/65 (25%)	8/161 (5%)
Total	1950		136/461 (29.5%)	146/1489 (9.8%)

[a] No prehospital defibrillation; all defibrillation achieved in hospital emergency department.

deliver five to ten times this number of lifesaves, particularly when combined with CPR by the citizen (Table 2) [24].

4. NONCONTROVERSY ABOUT PREHOSPITAL CORONARY CARE

The efficacy of prehospital ECC has repeatedly been called into question by workers in Nottingham in the United Kingdom [37–39]. Yet results in the USA, Canada and various countries in Europe including elsewhere in the United Kingdom, (Tables 2–4) vary remarkably with results of the sundry comparisons made in Nottingham among teams of physicians, nurses and paramedics, ordinary ambulance services, and treatment at home vs. treatment in hospital (Tables 2, 4). For example, CPR by itself as practiced in Winnipeg proved three times more effective than mobile intensive care as practised in Nottingham (Table 4). The experiments in emergency care in Nottingham were doomed to fail by features such as the provision of definitive prehospital services over 3 h after onset of symptoms of myocardial ischemia, the comparatively very low resuscitation rates by trained personnel (Tables 2, 4) and the insufficient number of patients for analysis [45]. Late entry of patients into the study and 2 h of prehospital intensive care before randomization into groups for treatment at home or in hospital excluded virtually all patients at greatest risk of ventricular fibrillation and sudden death and strongly supported the argument for prehospital coronary care [6]. Nagel's hypothesis that prehospital ECC contributed 5% to the reduction in coronary mortality in the USA appears low [46]. In Seattle, the yearly survival of 90–100 victims of prehospital ventricular fibrillation constitutes an estimated 10% reduction in community mortality [45]. In King County, Washington, paramedic service reduced community mortality by

8.4% [29]. A 15–20% reduction in community mortality occurred in the Virginia Piedmont [8] (Table 1, Figures 3, 5, 6). Resuscitation and defibrillation with long-term survival constitute measurable successful endpoints. Unfortunately, one can only estimate prevented fatalities, which certainly occur [21, 23] and doubtlessly make a significant contribution to the efficacy of prehospital coronary care [8].

5. COST AND BENEFITS OF PREHOSPITAL CORONARY CARE

Prehospital CPR and prehospital coronary care doubled our community's hospital coronary care unit admissions [5, 47]. Early hypothetical [48] and more recent practical [49] models of the impact of prehospital coronary care have been developed. Our calculation for adding prehospital coronary care to our extant ambulance service yielded a complementary benefit-to-cost ratio of 40:1 [8], but we did not budget for the costs and benefits of CPR by our citizens. The Seattle model incorporated the expense of CPR initiated by citizens [49]. We used Acton's assessment made in 1969 of $21,000 per 100 000 people for a livelihood lost to the community [48] to aid our calculation of actual benefits from the Seattle system. If the 1969 United States consumer price index (109.8) is adjusted upward to January 1981 (260.5), the saved livelihood is worth $49,823 per 100 000 people to the community. In 1976 the city of Seattle covered the cost of CPR training for 175 000 people amounting to $1.25 per citizen [50] totalling $220,000. The yearly 47 long-term saves of life (9.4 per 100 000 people) which reflect CPR by a citizen (Table 3) thus total $2.3 million or $468, 327 per 100 000 people. In 1982 the cost of educating the citizens of Seattle using the 1976 consumer price index (170.5) as a base would

Table 4. Influence of prehospital coronary care upon the community in Canada and Europe

Community	Yearly life-saves per 100 000 population		Ambulance personnel
Belfast	8.6	5.4[a] 3.2	Physician [40]
Brighton	4.4		Paramedic, EMT [41]
Edinburgh	3.4 & 5.7[b]		Physician [42]
Helsinki	3.0[c]		Physician [43]
Winnipeg	2.8[d]		EMT [36]
Dundee	2.6		Physician [44]
Nottingham	1.0		Physician [38]
Nottingham	1.0		Physician, para medic [37]

[a] Estimate of prevented ventricular fibrillation [21].

[b] 5.7 life-saves of persons aged 20–69 years per 100 000 people of this age group.

[c] 3.0 life-saves of persons aged <65 years per 100 000 people of all ages.

[d] Only basic life support (CPR) in prehospital phase; all defibrillation took place in hospital emergency department.

come to at least $ 336,129 or $ 7,152 per life saved. The complementary cost-to-benefit ratio ($ 336,129 : $ 2.3 million) thus crudely calculated is one dollar of expenditure for seven dollars worth of life saves for the city of Seattle. Consequently, citizen CPR favorably influenced $ 2.3 million worth of life saves, or just over half the annual Seattle life saves worth $ 4.5 million (Table 3). The benefits of these saved lives presumably justified the cost to the citizens of Seattle. The optimum distribution and number of citizens trained or retrained in CPR remains unknown. The lay person's skill in CPR decreases with time after training [51].

Fostering a citizenry trained to perform CPR seems a desirable goal in today's society given the frequency of sudden cardiac death and in view of the costs and benefits discussed above. Sufficient numbers of individuals in each neighborhood should learn CPR [52]. In families with a member at high risk of sudden cardiac death the spouse, off-spring and others should be taught CPR. The first responders to emergencies such as police, fire- and rescue squads and custodians should also learn CPR. Individuals working in factories, offices, stadia, theaters, concert-halls, and major transportation carriers and terminals should be trained in CPR.

6. MEDICAL CONTROL IN PREHOSPITAL CORONARY CARE

The physician must assume responsibility for individual and collective ECC of the patient in the prehospital phase if a high quality of service is to result. Medical control constitutes the direction by the physician of emergency care rendered by basic and intermediate EMTs, paramedics, nurses and physicians in the field and the direction of personnel involved in emergency communications such as ambulance dispatchers. The physician may function off-line through the use of protocols for treatment, review of cases, assessment of results, training programs for EMTs, paramedics, nurses and physicians, and community programs for citizen CPR. On-line medical control by the physician involves directing via radio or telephone the on-the-spot provider of emergency care before and during ambulance transport [53]. Only by aggressively functioning on- and off-line can the physician guarantee the community the highest quality of prehospital care with the greatest degree of favorable results for the coronary patient [54].

7. SUMMARY

Prehospital coronary care has proved an effective weapon against death and morbidity from ischemic heart disease in selected communities in the Virginia Piedmont, the United States, the United Kingdom and several other countries in Europe. As an emergency measure it appears to be cost-effective. Its efficacy triples when combined with CPR by citizens. Only stringent medical control by a physician can guarantee and maintain high quality of ECC. Thus the physician responsible for medical control remains the cornerstone of effective prehospital coronary care in the community.

REFERENCES

1. Pantridge JF, Geddes JS: Cardiac arrest after myocardial infarction. Lancet 1:807–808, 1966.
2. Pantridge JF, Geddes JS: A mobile intensive care unit in the management of myocardial infarction. Lancet 2:271–273, 1967.
3. Crampton RS, Stillerman R, Gascho JA, Aldrich RF, Hunter FP Jr, Harris RM Jr, McCormack RC: Prehospital coronary care in Charlottesville and Albemarle County. Virginia Med Month 99:1191–1196, 1972.
4. Crampton RS, Aldrich RF, Stillerman R, Gascho JA: Prehospital cardiopulmonary resuscitation in acute myocardial infarction. N Engl J Med 286:1320–1321, 1972.
5. Crampton RS, Aldrich RF, Gascho JA, Miles JR Jr, Stillerman R: Reduction of prehospital, ambulance, and community coronary death rates by the communitywide emergency cardiac care system. Am J Med 58:151–165, 1975.
6. Crampton R, Gascho J, Martin E: Taking coronary care to the patient. Lancet 1:1145–1146, 1978.
7. Crampton RS: Mobile coronary care: evaluation of efficiency. In: Acute Myocardial Infarction (Donoso E, Lipski J, eds.) pp. 27–36. New York, Stratton Intercontinental, 1978.
8. Crampton RS: Prehospital advanced cardiac life support: evaluation of a decade of experience. Top Emerg Med 1:27–36, 1980.
9. Nagel EL, Hirschman JC, Mayer PW, Dennis F: Telemetry of physiologic data: an aid to fire-rescue personnel in a metropolitan area. Southern Med J 61:598–601, 1968.
10. Nagel EL, Hirschman JC, Nussenfeld SR, Rankin D, Lundblad E: Telemetry – medical command in coronary and other mobile emergency care systems. JAMA 214:332–338, 1970.
11. Cobb LA, Conn RD, Samson WE, Philbin JE: Early experiences in the management of sudden death with a mobile intensive/coronary care unit. Circulation 41–42 (Suppl III): 144, 1970.
12. Baum RS, Alvarez H, Cobb LA: Survival after resuscitation from out-of-hospital ventricular fibrillation. Circulation 50:1231–1235, 1974.
13. Lewis RP, Fulkerson PK, Stang JM, Sampson KL, Dutko HJ: The Columbus emergency medical service system. Ohio State Med J 75:391–394, 1979.
14. Grace WJ, Chadbourn JA: The mobile coronary care unit. Dis Chest 55:452–455, 1969.
15. Lambrew CT: Experience in telemetry of the electrocardiogram to a base hospital. Heart Lung 3:756–764, 1974.
16. Lewis AJ, Criley JM: An integrated approach to acute coronary care. Circulation 50:203–205, 1974.
17. Criley JM, Lewis AJ, Ailshie GE: Mobile emergency care units. Implementation and justification. Adv Cardiol 15:9–24, 1975.
18. Edwards BW: Medical control and the volunteer rescue squad. J Emerg Med Services (JEMS) 6:38–42, 1981.
19. Oliver MF, Julian DG, Donald KW: Problems in evaluating coronary care units. Their responsibilities and their relation to the community. Am J Cardiol 20:465–474, 1967.
20. Stillerman R, Aldrich RF, McCormack RC, Crampton RS: Coronary artery disease (CAD) Death in a community before and after the advent of hospital coronary care units (CCU). Circulation 42(Suppl III): 202, 1970.
21. Pantridge JF: Mobile coronary care. Chest 58:229–234, 1970.
22. Aldrich RF, Stillerman R, McCormack RC, Crampton RS: Sudden coronary artery disease (CAD) Death in a community and the prospective role of mobile coronary care (MCCU). Circulation 42 (Suppl III):83, 1970.

23. Pantridge JF, Adgey AAJ, Geddes JS, Webb SW: The Acute Coronary Attack. New York: Grune & Stratton, 1975.
24. Thompson RG, Hallstrom AP, Cobb LA: Bystander-initiated cardiopulmonary resuscitation in the management of ventricular fibrillation. Ann Intern Med 90:737–740, 1979.
25. Lewis RP, Lanese RR, Stang JM, Chirikos TN, Keller MD, Warren JV: Reduction of mortality from prehospital myocardial infarction by prudent patient activation of mobile coronary care system. Am Heart J 103:123–130, 1982.
26. Keller MD: A study of the impact of mobile coronary care units. In: Emergency Medical Services Systems Research Projects. p. 74. Washington, DC, DHEW Publication No (PHS) 79-3220, 1979.
27. Hoffer EP: Emergency medical services. N Engl J Med 301:1118–1121, 1979.
28. Eisenberg MS, Bergner L, Hallstrom A: Out-of-hospital cardiac arrest: improved survival with paramedic services. Lancet 1:812–815, 1980.
29. Eisenberg M, Bergner L, Hallstrom A: Paramedic programs and out-of-hospital cardiac arrest. II. Impact on community mortality. Am J Publ Health 69:39–42, 1979.
30. Eisenberg MS, Copass MK, Hallstrom AP, Blake B, Bergner L, Short FA, Cobb LA: Treatment of out-of-hospital cardiac arrests with rapid defibrillation by emergency medical technicians. N Engl J Med 302:1379–1383, 1980.
31. Myerburg RJ, Conde CA, Sung RJ, Mayorga-Cortes A. Mallon SM, Sheps DS, Appel RA, Castellanos A: Clinical, electrophysiologic and hemodynamic profile of patients resuscitated from prehospital cardiac arrest. Am J Med 68:568–576, 1980.
32. Rockswold G, Sharma B, Ruiz E, Asinger R, Hodges M, Brieter M: Follow-up of 514 consecutive patients with cardiopulmonary arrest outside the hospital. J Am Coll Emerg Phys 8:216–220, 1979.
33. Lund I, Skulberg A. Cardiopulmonary resuscitation by lay people. Lancet 2:702–704, 1976.
34. Eisenberg MS, Bergner B, Hallstrom A: Paramedic programs and out-of-hospital cardiac arrest. I. Factors associated with successful resuscitation. Am J Publ Health 69:30–38, 1979.
35. Guzy PM, Pearce ML, Greenfield S, Beck L, McElroy CR: Effectiveness of citizen cardiopulmonary resuscitation during out-of-hospital emergencies in metropolitan Los Angeles. Circulation (Suppl II) 60:46, 1979.
36. Tweed WA, Bristow G, Donen N: Resuscitation from cardiac arrest: assessment of a system providing only basic life support outside of hospital. Can Med Assoc J 122:297–300, 1980.
37. Hampton JR, Dowling M, Nicholas C: Comparison of results from a cardiac ambulance manned by medical or non-medical personnel. Lancet 1:526–529, 1977.
38. Hill JD, Hampton JR, Mitchell JRA: A randomized trial of home-versus-hospital management for patients with suspected myocardial infarction. Lancet 1:837–841, 1978.
39. Hill JD, Hampton JR, Mitchell JRA: Home or hospital for myocardial infarction-who cares? Am Heart J 98:545–547, 1979.
40. Webb SW: Mobile coronary care. Lancet 1:559–560, 1974.
41. MacIntosh AF, Crabb ME, Grainger R, Williams JH, Chamberlain DA: The Brighton resuscitation ambulances; review of 40 consecutive survivors of out-of-hospital cardiac arrest. Br Med J 1:1115–1118, 1978.
42. Vetter NJ, Pocock S, Julian DG: Measuring the effect of a mobile coronary care unit upon the community. Br Heart J 41:418–425, 1979.
43. Siltanen P, Sundberg S, Hytönen I: Impact of a mobile coronary care unit on the sudden coronary mortality in a community. Acta Med Scand 205: 195–200, 1979.
44. McNeill GP, Bouchier IAD, Watson H: Mobile coronary care available to the general public. Lancet 1:975, 1979.
45. Adgey AAJ, Crampton RS: Hospital or home for acute myocardial infarction: another look at whether or not we should bother to care. Am Heart J 102:473–477, 1981.
46. Nagel EL: Prehospital care as a cause for coronary heart disease mortality decline. In: Proceedings of a Conference on the Decline in Coronary Heart Disease Mortality (Havlik RJ, Feinleib M, eds.) pp. 149–151. Washington DC: DHEW (NIH Publ No 79-1610), 1979.

47. Crampton RS, Michaelson SP, Aldrich RF, Gascho JA: Prehospital care for myocardial infarction. N Engl J Med 291:418, 1974.
48. Sidel VW, Acton J, Lown B: Models for the evaluation of prehospital coronary care. Am J Cardiol 24:674–688, 1969.
49. Hallstrom A, Eisenberg MS, Bergner L: Modeling the effectiveness and cost-effectiveness of an emergency service system. Soc Sci Med 15C; 13–17, 1981.
50. Cobb LA, Alvarez H, Copass MK: A rapid response system for out-of-hospital emergencies. Med Clin North Am 60:283–290, 1976.
51. Cobb LA, Hallstrom AP, Thompson RG, Mandel LP, Copass MK: Community cardiopulmonary resuscitation. Ann Rev Med 31:453–462, 1980.
52. McElroy CR: Citizen CPR: the role of the lay person in prehospital care. Top Emerg Med 1:37–46, 1980.
53. Committee on Emergency Medical Services: Medical control in emergency medical services systems. p. 4–5. Washington, DC: National Academy Press, 1981.
54. Pozen MW, D'Agostino RB, Sytkowski PA, Schneider RJ, Berezin MM, Brewer LH, Riggin RJ: Effectiveness of a prehospital medical control system: an analysis of the interaction between emergency room physician and paramedic. Circulation 63:442–447, 1981.

8. THE ROLE OF AMBULANCEMEN IN PRE-HOSPITAL CORONARY CARE

D.A. CHAMBERLAIN and C. STUDD

1. INTRODUCTION

Most of what is known of the natural history of coronary disease has been learnt in the short space of 20 years. Community studies made in this period have shown that approximately half of all deaths from acute events occur within an hour of the onset of any symptoms [1, 2]. The recognition of the fact that most early deaths were due to ventricular fibrillation and therefore potentially reversible led to the concept of coronary care units [3, 4], though the results were disappointing because few patients were admitted to hospital during the period of greatest risk [1]. Later evidence showed that many early deaths were instantaneous due to ventricular fibrillation without recent infarction, so that victims have no opportunity to seek help before the onset of circulatory arrest [5, 6].

The distinction between unheralded instantaneous arrhythmic cardiac death and early death following myocardial infarction cannot readily be made by pathologists. Thus today we are still uncertain of what proportion falls into either category, but from the point of view of practical therapy the categories share one feature which many still choose to ignore: conventional hospital treatment is unlikely to be made available in time to save the majority of people who die from electrical failure of the heart. The peak age for such deaths lies in the decade between 55 and 64 years [7].

If conventional measures are shown to be inappropriate to meet one of the greatest medical challenges of our time, then new concepts are needed. When the notion of delivering sophisticated hospital care to the patient suffering from an acute heart attack – using well-equipped coronary ambulances – was pioneered by the Belfast group in 1966 [8], most physicians and cardiologists were sceptical of its value. The tide of opinion is changing only slowly, and in Britain relatively few Health Districts are so equipped even 15 years later.

The reasons for the lack of progress are manifold, and scepticism may no longer be the most important of them. As originally conceived, coronary ambulances made use of medical and nursing personnel travelling either with the ambulance [8] or separately [9]. In this way a full range of treatment could be made available to the patient – drug therapy and pacing as well as defibrillation. This pattern could not be copied everywhere. Many hospitals are short-staffed, with essential hospital routines claiming all available time. A compromise solution was reached almost simultaneously and independently in several parts of the world. This came with the

Adgey, AAJ (ed): Acute phase of ischemic heart disease and myocardial infarction.
© *1982, Martinus Nijhoff, The Hague, Boston, London. ISBN-13: 978-94-009-7581-1*

realisation that much could be achieved without the direct intervention of medical and nursing staff.

Lown and Ruberman, in 1970, were among the first to suggest the possible role of paramedical personnel in mobile coronary care units [10]. In the same year Nagel [11] demonstrated that highly trained firemen could achieve fast response times for emergency care, and provide facilities for resuscitation at low cost by using telemetry to hospital-based physicians. The highly successful Seattle scheme also began in 1970 [12]. A group in Dublin reported in 1971 [13] the correction of ventricular fibrillation by ambulancemen who were not in telemetric communication with physicians.

Within a decade the practice of successful resuscitation outside hospital for patients with cardiac and other emergencies had become familiar in many parts of the world, and the role of paramedical personnel was gaining widespread acceptance. Though the concept of bringing advanced resuscitation techniques to the patient before hospital admission was pioneered in Europe both for accident cases [14] and for coronary emergencies [8], developments were most rapid in the United States. The lack of centrally organised free ambulance services was overcome in most areas by participation of Fire Departments.

In Europe pre-hospital coronary care remained principally the province of physicians. Paramedical training was slow to be adopted despite the availability of well-organised ambulance services. Early schemes included those in Brighton [15–17] and Copenhagen [18]. Similar programmes were soon set up in Australasia, notably in Melbourne [19] and later in Auckland [20]. Resuscitation by paramedical personnel was not yet widespread by the late 1970s, but it had become worldwide.

2. THE BRIGHTON EXPERIMENT

A coronary ambulance was established in Brighton in 1968 through the co-operation of the then Medical Officer of Health*, a senior hospital anaesthetist, and the chief ambulance officer. Despite the enthusiastic efforts which were made, manning the designated vehicle by hospital doctors or by general practitioners proved impracticable. Two years later one of the authors was appointed cardiologist in Brighton but did not participate in the scheme and remained sceptical of its potential value until faced in late 1970 by the unexpected collapse in ventricular fibrillation of a patient being visited at home. The coronary ambulance was summoned promptly. Though a series of mischances prevented a successful outcome in this case, two lessons were learnt which had important consequences: the new cardiologist accepted that defibrillation should not be confined to hospitals, and those who had struggled to maintain a service inadequately staffed by doctors agreed to accept as

---

* In Britain at that time the post of Medical Officer of Health was part of local government and carried wide responsibilities for community health.

an experiment the training of ambulancemen in advanced resuscitation techniques. The idea was thought to be novel though other similar schemes were by then already under way.

Six ambulancemen volunteered to enrol in a six-month course starting January 1971 and offered a service from July 1971 on [15]. The training which is provided for the ambulancemen, and the organisation of the system, have changed relatively little since that time.

The principles which determined the content of the course were the following:

1. Ambulancemen should be able to offer effective aid for all common life-threatening emergencies.
2. First aid measures should not include 'invasive' procedures.
3. Any drug treatment used should have a very wide margin of safety and should not cause local complications if incorrectly administered.
4. The course of instruction should be sufficiently comprehensive to give the ambulancemen the confidence that they would understand everything they were likely to see.
5. Ambulancemen should be competent to act on their own initiative without recourse to guidance by radio and telemetry.

An additional factor which determined the complexity of the syllabus in Brighton concerned logistics rather than principle: instruction to ambulancemen had to be given to a class which also comprised staff nurses undertaking a coronary care course. The syllabus had to meet the needs of both groups and was more comprehensive than was judged necessary for either group alone. In the event, the content of the course proved no obstacle for most participants, and experience has shown the benefits of a curriculum as broadly based as possible.

The principles which we followed nevertheless precluded some interventions important in resuscitation. For example the intravenous administration of sodium bicarbonate was forbidden because of the tissue necrosis which occurs if the solution is injected outside a vein. We now believe that constraints of this type are unnecessary and that ambulancemen trained to 'paramedic' standard should use skills commensurate with the tasks they face, without paying undue regard to what has previously been deemed appropriate or inappropriate for non-medical personnel, or to the risks of minor mishaps.

2.1. Training and proficiency

From the start the Brighton scheme was intended to provide a resuscitation rather than a cardiac service. There has been an emphasis, however, on cardiac problems which is due to its origins and which is reflected in the training programme. This may not be appropriate in areas with a higher incidence of trauma and a younger age structure within the community.

Initial selection for advanced training has been the responsibility of the training officer within the ambulance service: a pre-course examination offers the first hurdle for the prospective 'paramedic'. Instruction during the main hospital-based course is given over 24 lectures of 90 min each, plus one month full-time attachment to the cardiac unit. The syllabus covers the following: a brief revision of relevant anatomy; cardiovascular physiology; the natural history of coronary disease and its complications; clinical pharmacology of relevant drugs and the treatment of coronary disease; resuscitation procedures with emphasis on defibrillation; and electrocardiography, with special knowledge of arrhythmias to the standard expected of medical registrars. The examination after the course comprises a written section, together with an oral and practical evaluation of resuscitation skills. The pass rate of 70% is not always attained, but some of those who have failed the course have been permitted to take it again in their own time. Successful candidates are permitted to defibrillate patients in ventricular fibrillation or rapid ventricular tachycardia without supervision or advice by radio.

After at least six months practical experience, ambulancemen may apply for further instruction in endotracheal intubation, use of the oesophageal obturator airway, infusion techniques, and drug administration. The practical tests are stringent and may have to be taken repeatedly until competence is assured. These skills are then used at the discretion of the ambulancemen as circumstances dictate. The drugs which can be given intravenously at this stage comprise lignocaine and atropine for arrhythmias, dexamethasone to protect against cerebral ischaemia, and glucagon for hypoglycaemia.

Only recently has the use of intra-cardiac adrenaline been added to the ambulancemen's repertoire. Two years practical experience in resuscitation is a prerequisite, and the technique can be used only when other resuscitation efforts have been proved unsuccessful.

The logging of an Ambulance Emergency Incident report with electrocardiograms on each patient, which is examined by one of the Cardiology team, allows continuous assessment of 'paramedic' performance after training. A refresher period of five days taken annually within the hospital provides the opportunity for updating resuscitation skills and knowledge. Modifications to the incident report form are anticipated which will allow a closer monitoring of in-service proficiency and identify more accurately any deficiencies of knowledge and technical skills. This information will be used to tailor the refresher period to individual requirements as well as to provide the documentation often requested by 'paramedics' to confirm their continuing levels of proficiency.

2.2. Benefits of the Brighton scheme

The earliest benefit which accrued from the provision of resuscitation ambulances was a decrease in delay from onset of symptoms to arrival in hospital for patients with acute myocardial infarction. The median delay in the first half of 1971 was over 6 h; within 18 months this had decreased to about 2 h. The factors responsible were the increased awareness among general practitioners of the risks of early fatal arrhythmias, the conviction on the part of the patients that an ambulance would be sent on demand for victims of chest pain (though initial contact with the general practitioner was encouraged except in emergencies), and drastic curtailment of the 'red tape' required for admission – in effect the provision of an open-house policy for acute coronary care. Unfortunately, no recent progress has been made in further reducing admission delays which are almost entirely a result of patients' optimism about the likely course of an illness, together with their inappropriate consideration for practitioners and emergency services.

It is impossible to quantify the benefits of early admission. About 25 patients per year are defibrillated in hospital and discharged alive, whilst many others receive drug or pacemaker treatment for life-threatening arrhythmias which is likely to improve prognosis. Though most of the patients are admitted early in the course of their illnesses, we cannot say how many would not have survived without the accelerated admission made possible by the new emergency service.

Successful cardiac resuscitation outside hospital is more readily quantified and the benefits are therefore more convincing. In the first year of operation (1971–72) five patients were resuscitated and left hospital alive. By 1976 the annual number had reached 15 patients. Soon afterwards, the ambulance control rooms for several towns were amalgamated. Whilst this increased overall efficiency, response times worsened and successful resuscitation became unusual – for some time. Fortunately, greater experience with the new control system and greater participation by the general public in resuscitation procedures have reversed the trend and in the 12 months between November 1980 and October 1981 a total of 25 patients were resuscitated from out-of-hospital cardiac or respiratory arrest with survival to hospital discharge. These comprised 21 patients with ventricular fibrillation, 2 with asystole resulting from heart disease and 2 with respiratory arrest (one of whom also became asystolic).

2.3. The skills required for resuscitation

The records of the 25 resuscitated patients were examined in detail to discover the skills which were utilised to achieve a successful outcome. These are shown in Table 1.

The table provides incontrovertible evidence that ambulancemen who have had advanced training can save lives as a direct result of their interventions. In the 12-month series, 15 of the 25 patients (60%) had suffered apparent cardiac or respiratory arrest before the ambulance was summoned, and 16 (64%) had had an arrest before the ambulance arrived on the scene. Recovery from this situation in the absence of an on-the-spot capability for resuscitation hardly ever occurs. Moreover, little prospect for recovery would have existed for the remaining patients who developed ventricular fibrillation after arrival of the ambulance, for the long-term success rate of defibrillation depends critically on the time taken to restore co-

138

Table 1. The interventions which were required in 25 successful resuscitation attempts from November 1980 to October 1981

	Number of patients	Arrest occurred			Cardiac massage		Defib	Pacing	Intubation		Drug administration		
		Before amb. called	After amb. called	After amb. arrived	Community	Amb/men			Oesophageal obturator	Endotracheal	Ligno- caine	Atropine	Dexa- methasone
Ventricular fibrillation	21	11	1	9	8[a]	15	21	1	1	7	9	4	8
Asystole	3[c]	3	–	–	1[b]	2	1[d]	2	–	2	1	2	1
Respiratory arrest only	1	1	–	–	–	1	–	–	–	1	–	–	–
Overall totals	25	15	1	9	9	18	22	3	1	10	10	6	9

[a] In 4 cases given by an attending doctor.
[b] In 1 case given by an attending doctor.
[c] One incident caused by a primary respiratory arrest.
[d] Ventricular fibrillation supervened after treatment of asystole.

ordinated rhythm – effective cardiac massage is difficult to perform whilst patients are in transit.

The value of the other interventions is less easy to prove. Two patients had primary respiratory arrests: in these intubation and effective ventilation provided much better prospects for recovery than would inflation of the upper respiratory passages either by mouth-to-mouth breathing or by mechanical means. Moreover all ten patients who required intubation following cardiac arrest caused by ventricular fibrillation or asystole were severely anoxic and deeply unconscious before resuscitation was started and adequate oxygenation probably played a critical role in recovery.

We have only anecdotal evidence that the stabilisation of heart rhythm, often achieved by atropine and lignocaine, can make an important contribution to recovery. Dexamethasone was administered by ambulancemen to patients in whom cerebral anoxia was judged to be severe: we have found this prevents undue delay subsequently. Evidence for its value has been adduced from patients with head injury but its value in patients with cardiac arrest is uncertain as it is based on theoretical concepts rather than on evidence of clinical trials [21]. Thus some interventions which can be made by ambulancemen are demonstrably life-saving, whilst the value of others is more speculative.

We ourselves are convinced, however, that the repertoire of several skills in advanced resuscitation techniques all play a role in achieving long-term success for many of the patients with out-of-hospital cardiac arrest who can be reached within a few minutes. Claims have been made that the Brighton system has been tried and shown to be of little value; but in the Nottingham study, which is cited as evidence [22], the ambulancemen had a much less comprehensive training than was given in Brighton. The comparison of results may indicate the important role of supplementary skills which are often needed for the effective restoration of adequate cardiac function.

3. ADVANCED TRAINING IN BRITAIN: A STRUGGLE FOR ACCEPTANCE

The critics of advanced training of ambulancemen have had an important influence in slowing the development of schemes in Britain. In 1976, a DHSS (Department of Health and Social Security) memorandum stated that the value of coronary ambulance schemes had not been proved [23], and cautioned Area Health Authorities against permitting new developments in this field. All progress was halted at least temporarily. Though we believe that opinion within the DHSS has changed considerably in the light of further evidence and debate [24], the original injunction had not been withdrawn by 1981 and it is still used to justify prohibition of new schemes and to prevent developments in existing ones. Five years stagnation in a scheme that has provided obvious benefits has caused frustration to those providing the service, and has limited the degree of success which might have been achieved.

Table 2. Numbers of advanced trained ambulancemen in 5 area health authorities by 1981

Avon	50	trained personnel
Gloucestershire	65	trained personnel
Surrey	15	trained personnel
East Sussex	56	trained personnel
Oxford	40	trained personnel

3.1. The association of emergency medical technicians

The lack of official support has not checked all progress. Table 2 shows the list of ambulance services in Britain which have now accepted advanced training and provide appropriate services for the communities within their areas.

An important stimulus for the development of advanced training was the formation of the Association of Emergency Medical Technicians (AEMT) in 1978. The principle aims of the Association are to promote the continuation of advanced education for professional ambulance personnel in the United Kingdom, to promote the highest professional standards in the immediate care of casualties and acute medical emergencies, to foster international co-operation with similar groups worldwide, and to promote the professional status of advanced trained personnel. A national programme for advanced training has been developed: the course is divided into four stages, the last of which comprises full cardiopulmonary resuscitation techniques taught in a hospital environment. The first national registration examination will take place in September 1983. Candidates who pass all parts of the examination and achieve a satisfactory assessment rating will be issued with 'paramedic' certificates of proficiency; the intention is to provide a certificate of authorisation to undertake intravenous puncture and infusion, laryngoscopy, and endotracheal intubation, ECG monitoring, and electrical defibrillation. The degree of recognition which will be afforded by the ambulance authorities is still to be decided. At present (1981) AEMT has 590 registered members with advanced skills, and over 2000 associate members who are anxious to increase their expertise and achieve 'paramedic' status. Much of the training so far has been achieved on an ad hoc basis and relies on the goodwill and enthusiasm of local ambulance officers and medical practitioners. Advanced training must eventually depend on the widespread and certain availability of approved courses which reach carefully defined standards.

4. A CHOICE OF SYSTEMS

The role of ambulancemen in pre-hospital coronary care has evolved in diverse ways in response to local needs and prejudices, the opportunities for training, the availability of funds, and the various long-term aims of ambulance authorities. A standardised approach was neither to be expected nor to be desired until experience and results could identify methods which were proving successful, efficient, and cost-effective. In seeking to increase the involvement of ambulancemen in caring for patients with cardiac emergencies, four major and inter-related decisions must be made:

1. A choice is necessary between a system dedicated to the care of 'coronary' patients – in particular patients thought to have cardiac emergencies – and one designated to cater for all types of resuscitation.

2. Special ambulances can be held in readiness for certain types of emergency use, or alternatively a proportion (or all) first-line stretcher-bearing vehicles can be equipped for advanced resuscitation procedures.

3. The involvement of ambulancemen can be at several different levels. If pre-hospital care is to be provided principally by medical practitioners (who will usually be hospital-based) then ambulancemen will be trained only in a supportive role. More thorough training is necessary if care is to be provided by ambulancemen who are in contact only by telemetry with hospital medical staff [18]. Finally, comprehensive training must be given to 'paramedics' who carry on-the-spot responsibility for the diagnosis and treatment of emergencies.

4. Arguments can be adduced in favour of training only a proportion of 'front-line' ambulancemen or for training all who are capable of acquiring high proficiency skills.

Our experience in Brighton has convinced us that our policies relating to the first three issues are appropriate for widespread acceptance. The fourth point is still debatable in our view. We believe very strongly that dedicated ambulances are wasteful and inefficient. Such vehicles become obsolete before covering a fraction of their economical mileage. Of more importance, the quality of information received by ambulance control from the general public is often very poor, and reliable triage is impossible [25]. In many cases a control officer can do no more than suspect that an emergency of some type has occurred or may develop. That an ambulance is required will usually be certain, but for what purpose may not be predictable: possibilities include the assessment, and subsequent discussion with the general practitioner, of a patient who can be left at home, the transfer to hospital of a stretcher patient without complications, the skilled care of a patient with serious cardiac problems, or the need for resuscitation from other types of illnesses. Thus general purpose ambulances are best used for all known or suspected emergencies, and the vehicles should be equipped and staffed to provide immediate care for all who are seriously ill or injured.

The need for participation by medical practitioners is often impractical because of difficulties in staffing, and in any case is likely to introduce dangerous delay in response times. Telemetry places undue reliance on vulnerable technology, dictates that medical staff be immediately available in a given location, and also dilutes the value of on-the-spot appraisal of a situation which may be complex. Thus we favour most strongly the concept of comprehensive advanced training for ambulancemen in general purpose 'front-line' vehicles.

Opinions differ on the proportion of ambulancemen who should receive advanced training. The greater the numbers within any station the more comprehensive the cover which can be provided. Some argue that experience is diluted in this way and expertise is therefore more difficult to maintain. Approximately 6–8 men are required for every vehicle if all shifts are to be covered, with due allowance for holidays, illness, and the vagaries of rotas. If both crew members are to have advanced training, then 10 or 12 'paramedics' are needed for every equipped vehicle. This will involve most of those with duties on stretcher-bearing ambulances, and in busy areas enough emergencies will be handled to maintain adequate standards. Annual refresher courses of at least five working days within the hospital system should be mandatory however much experience is gained in the field.

In Britain, ambulances are used extensively for transport of sitting patients for hospital visits. Such work can be undertaken by personnel without advanced training. A two-tier system could therefore be evolved with a transport section distinct from an emergency section. Some objections, however, have been raised to this proposal from within the service.

5. ADVANCED TRAINING FOR CORONARY CARE: THE BALANCE SHEET

The advantages of advanced training for ambulancemen to 'paramedic' standards can easily be summarised. Skilled help and, if necessary, resuscitation measures can be provided with minimum delay if immediate liaison with medical practitioners is not required. Cost is small because no additional ambulances have to be bought and no additional medical staff have to be employed. Dedicated ambulances are not needed. The additional training given to ambulancemen provides added interest and satisfaction in the work which is done, and the quality of care tends to improve not only for those with critical emergencies but for all patients. This has a beneficial influence within an ambulance station which affects even those who have not received advanced training. Moreover the skills of the ambulanceman can develop with increasing experience over many years, whereas junior hospital doctors in the training grades (who are involved most directly with resuscitation) often leave before their potential has been realised.

There are disadvantages too in the provision of critical care by ambulancemen. Powerful analgesics such as opiates cannot be administered, the number of other drugs which can be given intravenously must be limited for reasons of safety, and up to now not all resuscitation techniques can be applied. In particular, pacing may be needed for cardiac emergencies, and this is not a practical possibility for the 'paramedic' whilst the pervenous placement of the pacing electrode is the only effective method. Other potential difficulties concern professional relationships. The formation of a group of ambulancemen who have 'paramedic' status can create problems within the ambulance service and problems in liaison with nurses within Accident and Emergency Departments. We have found, however, that problems can be avoided if advanced training is made widely available both to ambulancemen and to Accident Department nurses who also play a crucial role in the care of the critically ill.

6. THERAPEUTIC LIMITATIONS: CAN THEY BE RESOLVED?

Few would deny that well-trained medical practitioners can contribute more to the safety of the critically ill coronary patient than can well-trained ambulancemen; to believe otherwise would be to suggest the total irrelevance of the long years of medical training. The treatment of most emergencies in coronary care can, however, be taught relatively easily to those with aptitude and practical abilities.

Unfortunately most patients requiring out-of-hospital resuscitation have problems which cannot be overcome by simple measures. The treatment of cardiac arrest in a cardiac care unit usually involves only simple defibrillation, whereas a similar emergency remote from medical help is more likely to progress to a point at which defibrillation causes transient or refractory asystole and troublesome apnoea. Thus the ambulanceman, often working without skilled assistance, tends to face problems greater than those of the full cardiac arrest 'team' in hospital, and he is often faced with working under very adverse conditions. The limitations of therapy available to ambulancemen are considerable even when he deals with patients who have not suffered cardiac arrest. For example, a medical qualification is a legal prerequisite for the prescription of opiates in most countries, so that neither cardiac pain nor left ventricular failure can be treated by ambulancemen in the most appropriate manner. Most of the inherent difficulties can be overcome and the difference in the quality of care provided by ambulance and by medical staff does not need to be great.

Analgesia can be provided by ambulancemen in Britain in the form of Entonox (50% nitrous oxide, 50% oxygen). It is less familiar in other countries. The equipment, BOC Entonox apparatus (Figure 1) or Pneu Pac analgesia system (Figure 2), is designed to be self-administered, and regulations dictate that it should be used only in this way. The mask should fit snuggly and the valve opens automatically in response to a negative pressure of inspiration. Even under best conditions, sufficient air leaks around the mask to dilute considerably the concentration of nitrous oxide which is inhaled; but some alteration of consciousness should be apparent in about half a minute and effective analgesia is achieved in less than two minutes. Unfortunately those most in need of analgesia use the equipment least well. Patients with cardiac pain are frightened, and the fear is accentuated by the early effects of nitrous oxide; co-operation in achieving a seal at the mask is rarely adequate even initially and is not maintained by those in pain, especially as consciousness becomes slightly impaired. These difficulties can be lessened by adequately instructing patients before Entonox is used, by explaining that 'wooziness' is felt before pain is relieved and

144

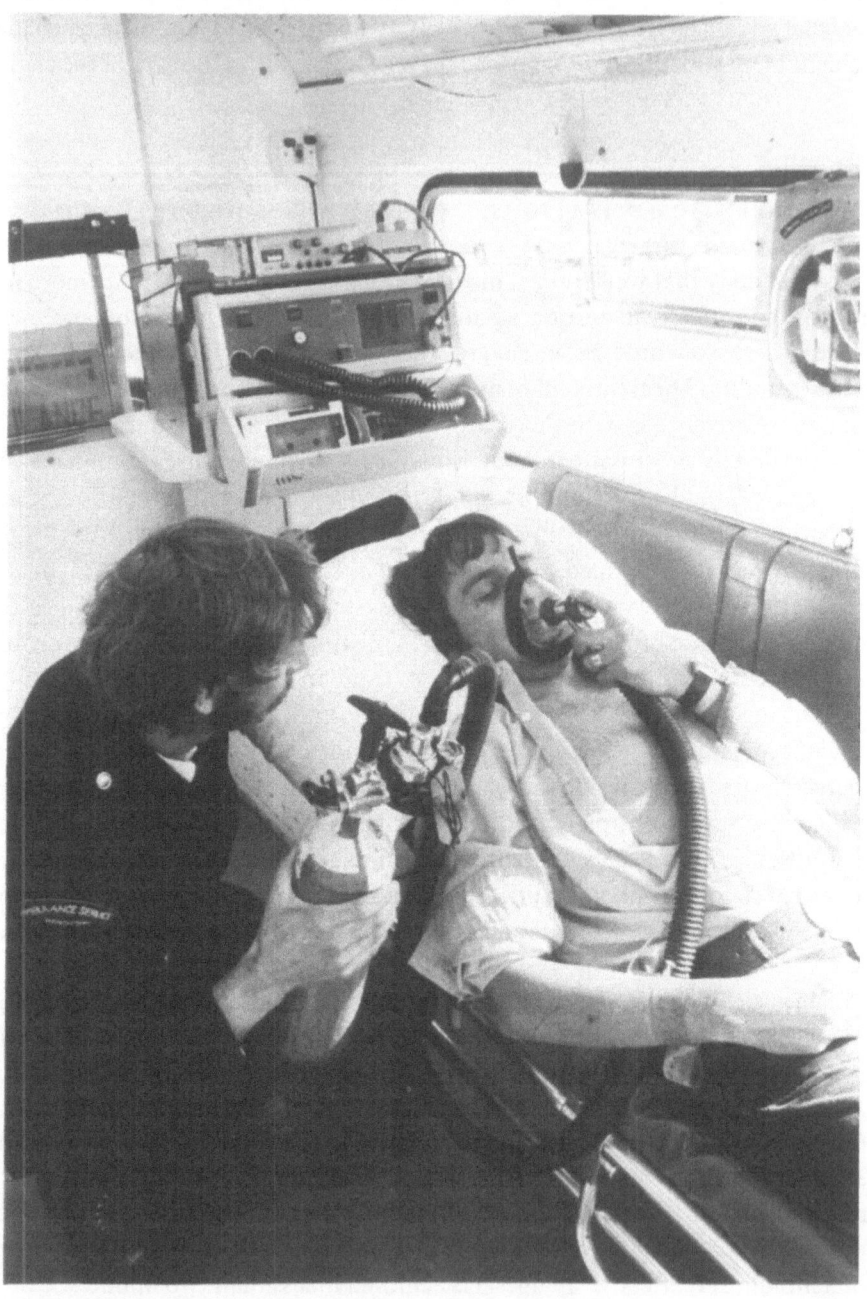

Figure 1. The BOC equipment for administration of nitrous oxide and oxygen analgesia.

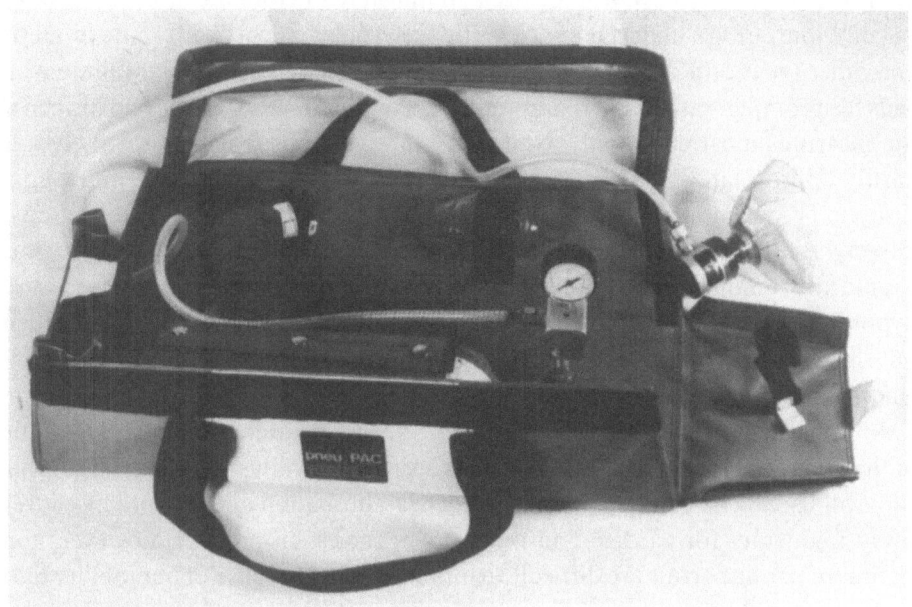

Figure 2. The Pneu Pac analgesia system for the administration of nitrous oxide and oxygen.

that treatment must be continued for several minutes for benefit to be noticed, and by assuring them that the mixture does not cause full loss of consciousness. Assistance for the patient in holding the mask in place seems sensible though usually this is not permitted. The flow of Entonox can be controlled by a valve which overrides the self-triggering mechanism. The use of this valve to obtain a constant flow of gas improves the inhaled concentration appreciably without causing danger. Those responsible for making and enforcing regulations may consider whether or not skilled ambulancemen should be constrained by rules designed more to deflect ill-informed criticism than to protect the well-being of the critically ill. Pain in myo-cardial infarction increases risk and probably increases the scale of necrosis because of the unfavourable haemodynamic effects of autonomic over-activity. The highest priority must be given to its relief. Entonox used to its best effect can produce useful analgesia even in myocardial infarction without important haemodynamic dis-turbance [26]. Its use by ambulancemen in the management of myocardial infarction is recommended; it should be delivered in an adequate concentration except for patients with chronic respiratory disease of a degree which renders high concentra-tions of oxygen dangerous. Other analgesics may be used by ambulancemen under 'blanket' instruction, but the safety, the rapid reversibility, and the potential efficacy of Entonox make it the agent of choice in the opinion of many who have experience in its use.

Left ventricular failure is a less common problem for advanced trained am-bulancemen than is cardiac pain. Its onset is less abrupt, so that medical help and appropriate therapy have usually been administered before the hazards of an ambulance journey are undertaken. Nevertheless, some patients with acute infarction and other types of heart disease do suffer unheralded left ventricular failure which calls for prompt treatment in the ambulance. At present reassurance and oxygen are the measures most commonly available – interventions which in themselves are hardly appropriate in case of a grave emergency. Whilst the use of intravenous furosemide by ambulancemen has advocates, the effect is relatively slow in onset. Glyceryl trinitrate lowers left ventricular filling pressure rapidly and we believe its use should be promoted for all patients with left ventricular failure who are not severely hypotensive. Sublingual administration may be difficult for very breathless patients but the glyceryl trinitrate sprays [27] now widely available in parts of Europe may lend themselves well to this purpose.

Apnoea can be countered much more effectively by intubation than by inflation of the upper respiratory passages. Ambulancemen providing pre-hospital coronary care will usually be competent in endotracheal intubation and will practise it relatively frequently for cardiac and other emergencies. In practice, however, some victims of cardiac arrest are difficult to intubate either because of immobility of the neck or, more commonly, because of the very cramped conditions under which emergency treatment has to be carried out. The oesophageal obturator airway [28] has proved of great value in such situations. It is passed with the neck flexed and enters the oesophagus – a technique achieved readily enough for other indications in gastric intubation. A balloon is inflated which seals the oesophagus, whilst air is forced through the upper tube through multiple holes placed just above the larynx. Ventilation is efficient provided the mouth and the nose are sealed (by a mask which is part of the equipment assembly), because the tongue cannot now obstruct the air passages. The oesophageal obturator can be left in place until endotracheal intubation is undertaken electively; this manoeuvre is aided rather than hindered by the presence of the first tube. Provided a choice of technique is available, intubation and effective ventilation are virtually always possible and can be achieved within seconds. This capability is not always found at emergencies within hospitals unless an anaesthetist is in attendance.

Pacing for asystole has been a deficiency in the management of patients with cardiac arrest by ambulancemen. Oesophageal electrodes offered a possible solution but ventricular 'capture' is not always possible. A solution has probably been achieved with the availability of the Pace-Aid (Cardiac Resuscitator Corporation, Oregon, USA). The equipment is shown in Figure 3. Ventricular activation is achieved 80 times per minute by stimuli of 50 to 150 mA between adhesive electrodes placed over the cardiac apex and the posterior mid thorax. This current is much lower than previously employed for external pacing, but is effective because the stimulus duration has been increased markedly from the conventional 2 ms to 20 ms. The electrode placement provides a low impedance pathway through the heart. During external pacing, some skeletal muscle stimulation occurs and the patient's arms and body may jerk. This can make palpation of the pulse more difficult but the

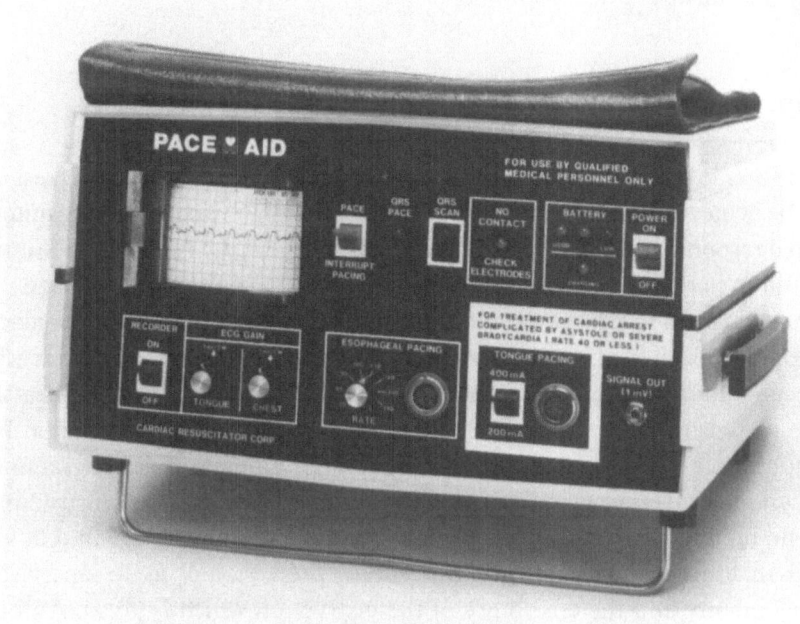

Figure 3. The Pace-Aid device for external pacing using either tongue-epigastrium electrode placement for ventricular stimulation or oesophageal placement for atrial stimulation.

device provides for an ECG and pulse display which can usually be interpreted despite muscle artefact. The Pace-Aid can – in its present form – be used for ventricular pacing only for unconscious or sedated patients. It can be used also for bi-polar oesophageal pacing to stimulate the atrium if atrio-ventricular conduction is intact. This is feasible even in conscious patients. External pacing has been used within our hospital for as long as 10 h in a successful attempt to resuscitate an asystolic patient with a tricuspid Starr-Edwards valve. Two of the three patients resuscitated from asystole by ambulancemen within the past year (see Table 1) also received external pacing which was probably life-saving.

The administration of intra-cardiac drugs by 'paramedics' has also been shown to be feasible and life-saving for patients with asystole or refractory ventricular fibrillation [29]. This has been added to the repertoire of skills used in Brighton and we believe the proportion of successful resuscitations will increase as a result.

In summary, greater experience in the use of ambulancemen to provide care of critically ill coronary patients has led to an increased emphasis on resuscitation techniques other than defibrillation. Moreover, technological advances have also helped to bridge the gap between what is available for medical practitioners and what can be achieved by 'paramedics'. The advantages of having hospital-based doctors in coronary care ambulances have lessened over the past 15 years, and it seems likely that this trend will continue.

7. COMMUNITY TRAINING: ANOTHER ROLE FOR AMBULANCEMEN?

Successful resuscitation for those who suffer from unheralded cardiac arrest is unlikely to be achieved unless skilled help is available within two or three minutes. Though rapid response times can be achieved routinely by Medic I vehicles in Seattle – and account in part for the excellent results in that city – most towns depend on ambulances which can reach few patients within five minutes after an emergency call. If an appreciable impact is to be made on the problem of sudden cardiac death, effective first aid must be available from within the community [30]. Again Seattle pointed the way, with more than 200 000 citizens having received instruction by 1978. A modest start has been made in Brighton to emulate this programme. Regular classes are given to groups of up to 40 people. Voluntary lay instructors each teach no more than four or five people around one training manikin, but we have found that the presence of an experienced 'professional' as a supervisor improves the quality and the credibility of the instruction which is given. Ambulancemen 'paramedics' fill this role admirably. Though only 14 000 of the community in Brighton have been instructed so far, direct intervention by those who have attended classes have already influenced favourably our success rate. An indirect impact has been evident as well, reflected in more prompt alerting of the ambulances in response to actual or potential emergencies; this is a result of better understanding within the community of the problems and natural history of acute coronary disease. We believe that the provision of a resuscitation ambulance system and the provision of community instruction in cardiopulmonary resuscitation should go hand-in-hand. Good results from attempted resuscitation cannot be achieved by either intervention alone. The advanced training of ambulancemen offers an excellent method of manning the rescue ambulances, and also provides the backbone for the corps of instructors needed to educate the community.

ACKNOWLEDGEMENTS

We thank Mr R Grainger, Chief Ambulance Officer whose continuing participation makes the scheme possible. We also thank Mrs E. Quinn, Research Assistant, who has maintained records with the greatest care.

REFERENCES

1. Smyllie HC, Taylor MP, Cunninghame-Green RA: Acute myocardial infarction in Doncaster II – Delays in admission and survival. Br Med J 1:34–36, 1972.

2. Kinlen LJ: Incidence and presentation of myocardial infarction in an English community. Br Heart J 35:616–622, 1973.

3. Brown KWG, MacMillan RL, Forbath N, Mel'grano F, Scott JW: Coronary unit: an intensive-care centre for acute myocardial infarction. Lancet 2:349–352, 1963.

4. Day HW: Preliminary studies of an acute coronary care area. J Lancet (Minneapolis) 83:53–55, 1963.

5. Liberthson RR, Nagel EL, Hirschman JC, Nussenfeld SR: Prehospital ventricular defibrillation: prognosis and follow-up course. N Engl J Med 291:317–321, 1974.

6. Cobb LA, Baum RS, Alvarez H, Schaffer WA: Resuscitation from out-of-hospital ventricular fibrillation: 4 years follow-up. Circulation 52 Suppl III:223–228, 1975.

7. Kannel WB, Doyle JT, McNamara PM, Quickenton P, Gordon T: Precursors of sudden coronary death: factors related to the incidence of sudden death. Circulation 51:606–613, 1975.

8. Pantridge JF, Geddes JS: A mobile intensive care unit in the management of myocardial infarction. Lancet 2:271–273, 1967.

9. Barber JM, Boyle DMcC, Chaturvedi NC, Gamble J, Groves DHM, Millar DS, Shivalingappa G, Walsh MJ, Wilson HK: Mobile coronary care. Lancet 2:133–134, 1970.

10. Lown B, Ruberman W: The concept of precoronary care. Mod Concepts Cardiovasc Dis 39:97–102, 1970.

11. Nagel EL, Hirschman JC, Nussenfeld SR, Rankin D, Lundblad E: Telemetry - medical command in coronary and other mobile emergency care systems. JAMA 214:332–338, 1970.

12. Baum RS, Alvarez H, Cobb LA: Survival after resuscitation from out-of-hospital ventricular fibrillation. Circulation 50:1231–1235, 1974.

13. Gearty GF, Hickey N, Bourke GJ, Mulcahy R: Pre-hospital coronary care service. Br Med J 3:33–35, 1971.

14. Collins J: Organization and function of an accident flying squad. Br Med J 2:578–580, 1966.

15. White NM, Parker WS, Binning RA, Kimber ER, Ead HW, Chamberlain DA: Mobile coronary care provided by ambulance personnel. Br Med J 3:618–622, 1973.

16. Briggs RS, Brown PM, Crabb ME, Cox TJ, Ead HW, Hawkes RA, Jequier PW, Southall DP, Grainger R, Williams JH, Chamberlain DA: The Brighton resuscitation ambulances: a continuing experiment in prehospital care by ambulance staff. Br Med J 2:1161–1165, 1976.

17. Mackintosh AF, Crabb ME, Grainger R, Williams JH, Chamberlain DA: The Brighton resuscitation ambulances: review of 40 consecutive survivors of out-of-hospital cardiac arrest. Br Med J 1:1115–1118, 1978.

18. Pederson A: Ambulance, hjertestop, og telemetri. Ugeskr Laeger 132:785–787, 1970.

19. Luxton M, Peter T, Harper R, Hunt D, Sloman G: Establishment of the Melbourne mobile intensive care service. Med J Aust 1:612–615, 1975.

20. Norris RM: Life threatening cardiac arrhythmias: management outside hospital. Patient Management: 17–25, August 1979.

21. Anonymous: Anoxic-ischaemic brain injury. Br Med J 3:73–74, 1974.

22. Hampton JR, Nicholas C: Randomized trial of a mobile coronary care unit for emergency calls. Br Med J 1:1118–1121, 1978.

23. Health Notice HN (76) 204. Health Services Development. Ambulance Service: Advanced training for ambulancemen. DHSS. November 1976.

24. The Ambulance Service of the Future. National Health Service Training and Studies Centre, Harrogate. DHSS. June 1979.

25. Cameron M, Wilkinson F, Hampton JR: Follow-up of emergency ambulance calls in Nottingham: implications for coronary ambulance service. Br Med J 1:384–386, 1975.

26. Thornton JA, Fleming JS, Goldberg AD, Baird D: Cardiovascular effects of 50% nitrous oxide and 50% oxygen mixture. Anaesthesia 28:484–489, 1973.

27. Chevigne M, Collignon P, Kulbertus H: Haemodynamic response to nitroglycerin in spray at rest and during exercise in sitting position. Unpublished observations.

28. Don Michael TA: The esophageal obturator airway. A critique. JAMA 246:1098–1101, 1981.

29. Amey BD, Harrison EE, Staub EJ, McLeod M: Paramedic use of intracardiac medications in prehospital sudden cardiac death. JACEP 7:130–134, 1978.
30. Lund I, Skulberg A: Cardiopulmonary resuscitation by lay people. Lancet 2:702–704, 1976.

9. PRE-HOSPITAL EMERGENCY CARE IN THE USA: EFFECTIVENESS OF PARAMEDIC AND EMERGENCY MEDICAL TECHNICIAN UNITS

MICKEY S. EISENBERG and THOMAS HEARNE

1. INTRODUCTION

A quiet revolution has occurred in the delivery of out-of-hospital emergency medical care. It is a revolution that is probably invisible to the majority of citizens. Nevertheless, significant changes have occurred in the organization and technology of emergency medical services. What once would be considered acceptable treatment for medical emergencies is now being considered neglect. When once emergency care was provided by ambulance attendants and firefighters with often no formal medical training, care is now provided by highly trained emergency medical technicians and paramedics. When once vehicles responded without oxygen or other medical supplies and were used as hearses between ambulance runs, mobile medical intensive care units now bring hospital capability directly to the scene of an emergency.

This chapter will briefly recount the milestones in the history of emergency medical services in the U.S. over the last 15 years, a period when pre-hospital emergency care has moved from neglect to sophisticated medical care. The paper also will describe the effectiveness of paramedic and emergency medical technician units in the United States.

2. HISTORY

The initial impetus for improving out-of-hospital emergency care occurred in part from several national reports and from increasing public recognition of the vast numbers dying on highways [1]. The National Academy of Sciences issued a report in 1966 which labelled trauma as the 'neglected disease of modern society' [2].

In 1966 the federal government passed the National Highway Safety Act which provided for concerted efforts to train personnel and equip ambulances with appropriate instruments for dealing with trauma. Responsibility was assigned to the U.S. Department of Transportation (DOT) to set guidelines for emergency medical services and disburse funds for the purchase of ambulances, installation of communication systems, and development and support of emergency medical technician training programs. A major achievement of the National Highway Safety Act was the establishment of a training program for ambulance and emergency

Adgey, AAJ (ed): Acute phase of ischemic heart disease and myocardial infarction.
© *1982, Martinus Nijhoff, The Hague, Boston, London. ISBN-13: 978-94-009-7581-1*

personnel in basic life support techniques. The 81 hour course of instruction (developed in conjunction with the National Academy of Sciences and the American Academy of Orthopedic Surgeons) was intended to teach emergency care fundamentals such as maintenance of oral airway, control of external hemorrhage, administration of cardiopulmonary resuscitation, and immobilization of the patient with multiple injuries prior to transport to hospital [3]. The graduate of the training was designated an emergency medical technician (EMT). It is estimated that 300 000 individuals have been certified as EMT's in the United States which represents the majority of ambulance and emergency personnel providing out-of-hospital care. Certification is usually valid for three years with refresher courses and recertification examinations then required.

During the 1960's the emphasis of prehospital emergency care was on the provision of basic life support (cardiopulmonary resuscitation (CPR), airway management, and hemorrhage control) in the initial treatment of trauma. The underlying premise of this service was that the emergency medical care as delivered by EMT's could perhaps save lives from trauma and, if nothing else, would at least not harm individuals prior to arriving at the hospital for definitive care. The aim was to provide quality first aid at the scene and rush the patient to the hospital for definitive care. The EMT curriculum placed relatively little emphasis on treatment of medical emergencies at the scene.

During the late 1960's and 1970's a more sophisticated type of out-of-hospital emergency care emerged. The seminal work of Drs. Pantridge and Geddes in Belfast, Ireland showed that emergency coronary care could be delivered with a mobile unit directly at the scene of a cardiac emergency [4, 5].

The development of out-of-hospital coronary care was also aided by technological innovations including miniaturization of defibrillation equipment, improved cardiac monitoring, remote telemetry and the availability of antiarrhythmic medications. The first mobile intensive care unit in the United States, which began in New York City, was staffed by physicians and nurses (patterned after the Belfast unit set up by Pantridge) and provided antiarrhythmic drugs, as well as defibrillation for cardiac arrest due to ventricular fibrillation [6]. Early mobile intensive care unit programs in the United States were staffed with physicians and nurses. This pattern of staffing changed when it was demonstrated that specially trained lay personnel could provide equivalent emergency care and successfully stabilize patients at the scene using advanced medical techniques. By the second half of the seventies, physician and nurse staffing was replaced by specially trained individuals known as paramedics. Miami, Seattle, Los Angeles, Pittsburgh and Long Island, New York and other cities pioneered this concept of specially trained individuals known as paramedics. Paramedics were initially trained to deal with acute out-of-hospital coronary problems. Skills allowing paramedics to treat other medical and traumatic emergencies such as burns, injuries, drug and alcohol overdose, and others were subsequently added. Although each program established various training courses emphasizing different skills, what they all had in common was the ability of the highly trained paramedic to treat out-of-hospital patients using definitive procedures. While the training encompassed many types of medical and traumatic emergencies, major emphasis was placed on the treatment of myocardial infarction and specifically cardiac arrest. Each program had a slightly different administrative arrangement. In some cities the program was operated by the local fire department. In others a separate public agency was established, and in still others private ambulance companies provided paramedic services [7].

The development of paramedic programs occurred slowly during the early 70's and only a handful of cities operated these programs. In 1973, however, in the United States a major boost occurred with the passage of federal legislation. That year Congress passed the Emergency Medical Services Systems (EMSS) Act. This act created an Office of Emergency Medical Services within the Department of Health, Education and Welfare. Funding for a three-year period was $ 185 million. The act assisted in the definition of an integrated systems approach to out-of-hospital emergency care and established regional Emergency Medical Service (EMS) systems throughout the country. The act defined 15 elements of an emergency medical service system: manpower, training, communications, transportation, facilities, critical care units, public safety agencies, consumer participation, accessibility to care, transfer of patient, standardized patient record-keeping, public information and education, independent review and evaluation, disaster linkages, and mutual aid agreements [1]. The program identified 300 regions countrywide suitable for development of emergency systems. Most importantly for the development of paramedic programs, the act funnelled millions of dollars into the training of paramedics and the establishment of such programs. The EMSS act was renewed in 1976 and again in 1979. By 1980, 10 000 paramedics had been trained.

In addition to federal legislation, an important source of funding for the development of regional emergency dispatch centers using a 3-digit telephone access number (911) has been the Robert Wood Johnson Foundation. Public interest in emergency services has been due to the popularization of paramedic services on television shows (a popular weekly series known as 'Emergency' described the heroics of Los Angeles paramedics). Other developments which have heightened interest in emergency care have been the establishment of specialty boards in emergency medicine and residency training programs.

As opposed to emergency medical technicians who use a standardized training format, recommendations for paramedic training have only recently been formulated [8]. Consequently, each local community provides different training for paramedics and the amount of training may vary from several hundred to 1500 hours.

When paramedic services began, there was a clear distinction between the medical capabilities of the emergency medical technician and those of the paramedic. The emergency medical technician provided basic life support and the paramedic could provide some types of definitive care as a result of special training in defibrillation, endotracheal intubation, and administration of emergency medications. In recent years this distinction has become blurred as intermediate level emergency personnel

154

Table 1. Names, synonyms and skills of EMT's, intermediate personnel and paramedics

	EMT	EMT-I.V.	EMT-Airway	EMT-Defib	Paramedic
Synonyms	EMT Basic EMT-1	EMT-2	EMT-3		EMT-P EMT-4
Training period	81 hours	Approx. 200 h	Approx. 300 h	9 h	Approx. 400–1500 h
Skills	CPR	Establishing I.V. Line	Providing endotracheal or esophageal obturator airway control	Defibrillation	Advanced cardiac and trauma life support

have been trained to provide emergency services. Some of these intermediate level personnel include EMT's trained in intubation, or in the administration of intravenous fluids, or in defibrillation. The effectiveness of these intermediate level EMT's in improving patient survival has generally not yet been well established. One exception are EMT's trained in defibrillation, where initial studies show substantial increases in survival of patients with ventricular fibrillation. In Table 1 the names, synonyms, and skills of the intermediate personnel as well as EMT's and paramedics are listed. In this chapter, unless otherwise specified, EMT will refer to an EMT who has received only the basic 81-hour course of instruction and paramedic will refer to an individual capable of delivering advanced cardiac life support directly at the scene of an emergency. Similarly, the terms 'emergency medical technician services' and 'paramedic services' will refer to care provided by the above individuals. Unfortunately, there is a disparity of names applied to advanced emergency care programs often called paramedic services. They are also known by terms descriptive of their primary treatment focus or the training level of the personnel, for example, Advanced Cardiac Life Support, Mobile Coronary Care Unit, EMT Defibrillation, etc. It is noteworthy that emergency medical technician personnel now provide basic emergency medical care in most fire departments and ambulance companies. Most of the population requesting emergency help will have an individual trained to the level of EMT provide the care. In addition, many urban and suburban communities have intermediate emergency medical technicians and/or paramedics providing emergency care. Some communities, such as Seattle, Wash., have combined EMT and paramedic services into a tiered response system. The first responding unit is a fire department vehicle staffed with EMT's and the second unit, usually arriving several minutes later, is staffed with paramedics. Such a tiered response allows rapid initiation of basic life support (CPR) followed by advanced life support.

3. EFFECTIVENESS

Despite the historical roots of emergency medical services in the management of trauma, there have been no studies which demonstrate a benefit of this service in the treatment of trauma. While some benefits undoubtedly occur on a case by case basis, methodologic difficulties in performing such studies have precluded definitive statements concerning the effectiveness of EMS in treating trauma on a community wide basis. On the other hand, there have been studies demonstrating effectiveness of paramedic and emergency medical technician units in the treatment of cardiac emergencies, specifically cardiac arrest.

3.1. Evidence of effectiveness

Demonstration of effectiveness in the management of cardiac arrest when treated by paramedics comes from numerous case series. In Table 2, major studies reporting 26 or more attempted resuscitations by paramedic programs are listed [9–30]. Each study appeared in a refereed U.S. professional medical journal. Pre-hospital paramedic programs are defined as those having the capability of providing definitive care for cardiac arrest at the scene. 'Case definition' refers to the criteria necessary for the inclusion of a specific case in the study. 'Methodology' refers to the primary method of inquiry which characterizes each study, for example, type of study (descriptive, analytic, retrospective, prospective, quasi-experimental), type of groups in study design (control groups, comparison groups, cohort groups), size and characteristics of the study population or sample. The 15 locations shown in Table 2 geographically represent the country except that the locations are predominantly urban or suburban (some suburban areas include rural components). This predominant urban focus reflects the fact that most paramedic programs are found in these settings.

In Table 2 the outcome data for cardiac resuscitations are shown. Listed are the number of attempted resuscitations as well as the number of patients admitted to hospital and discharged alive from hospital. The range of attempted resuscitations is large, 26 to 1106. The number in each study is partially a function of the case definition, methods, and study duration. The percentage of cardiac arrest patients admitted varies between 17% and 65% (mean 38%) and the percentage of patients discharged alive varies from 3.5 to 31% (mean 18%).

It must be pointed out that while most of the studies report outcomes of cardiac arrest from all etiologies, some studies do not distinguish cardiac arrest due to heart disease from that due to non-heart disease or trauma [20, 24, 28]. Other studies report resuscitation outcomes primarily from patients with underlying ischemic heart disease [9, 10, 13, 16–18]. Some studies report cardiac arrest in patients with ventricular fibrillation on arrival of the paramedic units [21, 22, 25–27]. In two studies outcome data are reported according to a number of etiologies and in a variety of modes [11, 12]. Four distinct case definitions are used in the studies: 1)

Table 2. Cardiac arrest outcome studies: case definitions, methodological characteristics and summary outcome data

Location	Case definition	Methodology	Attempted Resuscitations	Patients admitted[a]	Patients discharged[a]	Post-discharge survival
1. Baltimore, MD (9, 10)	Suspected acute ischemic heart disease receiving ECG telemetry and therapy and ambulance transport.	22-month retrospective study of 7,654 patients transported, 179 of whom had telemetered ECGs and ASHD comparison groups.	28	12 (42.8%)[b]	6 (21.4%)	6 at 3 months
2. Charlottesville, VA (11, 12)	Cardiac arrest due to acute myocardial infarction.	31-month, before and after study of 460 paramedic responses. Cross-community comparison.	26	17 (65.4%)[b]	8 (30.8%)	Not recorded
3. Cincinnati, OH (13)	Cardiac arrests managed by paramedics; all etiologies.	1 year prospective study. No control group.	147	48 (32.7%)	22 (15.0%)	Not recorded
4. Columbus, OH (14)	Cardiac arrests, all etiologies.	Retrospective comparison study of patients treated by physician-manned or EMT-manned MCCU.	71[c] 61[d]	34 (48.0%)[b] 32 (52.5%)	16 (22.5%) 15 (24.6%)	Not recorded
5. Irvine, CA (15)	Cardiac arrests occurring after paramedic arrival; etiology uncertain, mainly primary heart disease.	15 month retrospective study. Detailed outcome of 26 cases; no control groups.	26	10 (38.5%)[b,e]	6 (23.1%)[e]	Not recorded
6. King County, WA (16-18)	Cardiac arrests due to primary heart disease.	Prospective, 3 year quasi-experimental study; control groups	301[f] 156[g]	51[b] (17%) 61[b] (39%)	18[b] (6%) 42[b] (27%)	17-month follow-up.

157

Location	Population	Study	N			Follow-up
7. Lincoln, NB (19)	Cardiac arrests; all etiologies.	Descriptive summary of Lincoln system over 30 months; no control groups.	169	—	35 (20.7%)[b]	Not recorded
8. Los Angeles, CA (20)	Cardiac arrest; all etiologies.	Summary of 3-year pilot program; general and summary outcome data; no control groups.	186	85 (45.7%)[b]	35 (18.8%)[b]	Not recorded
9. Miami, FL (21, 22)	Patients in ventricular fibrillation.	Retrospective historical study; no control group.	301 (VF)	101 (33.6%)	42 (14.0%)	Mean survival about 13 months
10. Minneapolis, MN (23)	Cardiac arrest; all etiologies.	2-year prospective study of 514 consecutive patients with follow-up; no control group.	514	170 (33.0%)	83 (16.0%)	Of 49 ambulatory patients, 15% died first year, 50% second year
11. Portland, OR (24)	Cardiac arrest; all etiologies.	Descriptive summary of Portland system over a 4-year period; no control group.	210	81 (38.6%)[b,h]	38 (18.1%)[b]	Not recorded
12. Seattle, WA (25–27)	Patients in ventricular fibrillation.	Prospective 4-year clinical study; compares outcomes for 2 periods; no control groups.	511 (VF)[i] 595 (VF)[j]	174 (34.0%)[b] 256 (43.0%)[b]	56 (11.0%)[b] 137 (23.0%)[b]	4-year follow-up for patients with AMI or Primary VF
13. Stanford, CA (28)	Consecutive cardiac arrest patients treated in emergency department following prehospital arrest.	2-year prospective study dealing with guidelines for resuscitations; no control group.	198	47 (23.7%)	7 (3.5%)	7 alive at 2 months

Table 2. (Cont.)

Location	Case definition	Methodology	Attempted Resuscitations	Patients admitted[a]	Patients discharged[a]	Post-discharge survival
14. Tampa, FL (29)	Patients in ventricular fibrillation.	Retrospective and prospective study using criteria for Sudden Death; no control group.	296 (VF)	—	34 (11.5%)	Survival reported by NYHA functional class
15. Torrance, CA (30)	All consecutive patients transported; all etiologies.	11-month retrospective study; case review of appropriate paramedic response; no control group.	112	24 (22%)	15 (13.4%)[b]	Not recorded

(Adapted from Eisenberg M, Bergner L, Hearne T: Out-of-hospital cardiac arrest: a review of major studies and a proposed uniform reporting system. Am J Public Health 70:236–240, 1980 reprinted with permission of publisher.).

[a] Percentages are expressed in terms of total attempted resuscitations reported.
[b] Figures not provided in this form but calculable from data given.
[c] Outcomes reported for Heartmobile.
[d] Outcomes reported for Medic unit.
[e] Includes one person admitted and transferred from another hospital.
[f] Outcomes reported for EMT service.
[g] Outcomes reported for paramedic service.
[h] Includes both patients alive in emergency rooms and those admitted to hospital.
[i] Resuscitation reported for first 2-year period.
[j] Resuscitation recorded for second 2-year period.

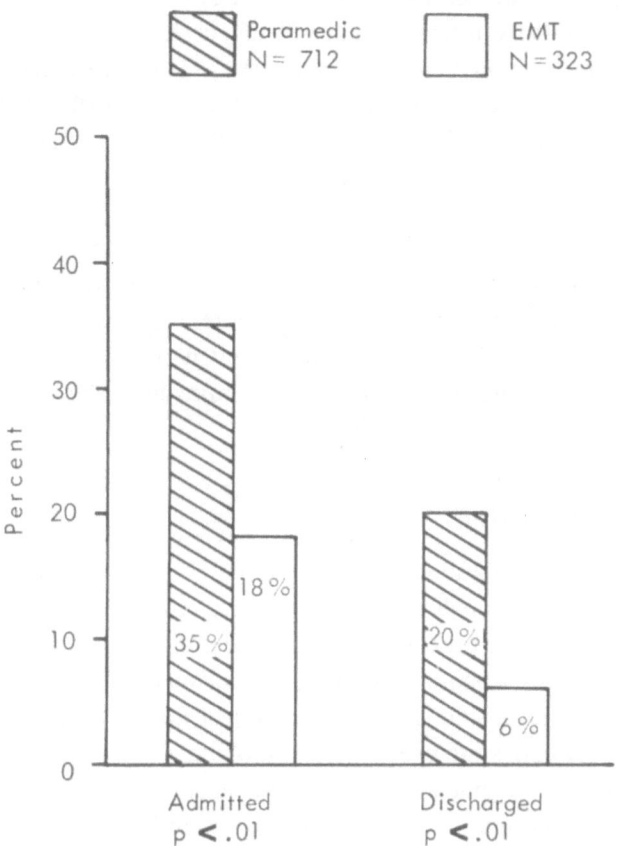

Figure 1. Type of service and outcome of cardiac arrests due to heart disease in King County, Washington.

cardiac arrest due to any etiology; 2) cardiac arrest due to heart disease; 3) ventricular fibrillation on arrival; and 4) cardiac arrest after paramedic arrival.

The studies show considerable variation in purpose and methodologic characteristics and reported outcomes. Some studies reported attempted resuscitations only as part of a large descriptive summary of paramedic services [11, 12, 19]. Others report outcomes in the context of improving paramedic response or providing objective criteria for deciding when resuscitation should be discontinued or not attempted [15], and still others emphasize outcomes as evaluative measures of paramedic systems [16–18, 21, 22, 25–27, 31]. While all of the studies fail to utilize experimental design, in part due to the difficulty of doing randomized studies with human populations, one study did utilize a quasi-experimental design with control groups [16–18]. This study, from King County, Wash, had the opportunity to compare emergency medical technician care and paramedic care. The study demonstrated that paramedics tripled the survival rate from cardiac arrest compared to emergency medical technician care. Discharge rates jumped from 6 to 20% following initiation of paramedic services. In Figure 1 the improvement in the outcome of cardiac arrest patients from King County, Wash, is shown.

The above studies demonstrate the effectiveness of paramedic services for out-of-hospital cardiac arrest. There is little doubt that an individual with an out-of-hospital cardiac arrest would have no chance of survival if not treated by emergency medical personnel. What is not clear, however, is the relationship between the life-saving benefit of paramedics and that of the emergency medical technicians. The study reported from King County, Wash suggests a two- to threefold improvement in survival rates. This study, of course, may be applicable only to that area and different communities may have a smaller or greater improvement. It is dangerous to extrapolate one study to an entire nation, but it seems safe to conclude that paramedics save lives and appear to save far more lives than can be saved by emergency medical technicians [16–18].

3.2. Reasons for effectiveness

Many of the reasons why paramedic programs save lives have to do with the manner in which the emergency medical system operates. Clearly, factors such as easy telephone access to emergency care, highly trained individuals, sophisticated care in emergency room and coronary care units, arrangements for communication between paramedics and hospitals, all have an effect on providing an efficient and effective emergency care system. Specifically looking at the event of cardiac arrest, there are well-defined reasons why an individual may live or die following collapse. Essentially, the factors determining survival or death following cardiac arrest can be divided into two groups: 1) fate factors, and 2) system factors.

Fate factors include clinical circumstances as well as circumstances at the time of collapse. Fate factors lie outside the control of the EMS system. For example, a massive myocardial infarction involving greater than 40% of the myocardium would not be compatible with life no matter what kind of emergency care system existed. Also important is the cardiac rhythm; patients in ventricular fibrillation may be successfully resuscitated if care is provided rapidly enough. On the other hand, patients in other cardiac rhythms have virtually no likelihood of survival. Another factor is whether the cardiac arrest was witnessed or unwitnessed. Persons whose collapse is witnessed are far more likely to survive cardiac arrest than are those whose collapse is not witnessed.

System factors are those over which the EMT's system has direct influence; they include the type of emergency service provided. If care is provided by paramedics, there is a two- to threefold increase in likelihood of survival compared to EMT programs. Other system factors include the time from collapse to initiation of cardiopulmonary resuscitation and the time from collapse to provision of definitive care. As seen in Figure 2, if cardiopulmonary resuscitation is initiated rapidly 28% of patients are discharged compared to 13% of patients if CPR is delayed beyond 4 min. Similarly, if definitive care is provided in less than 6 min, 36% of patients are

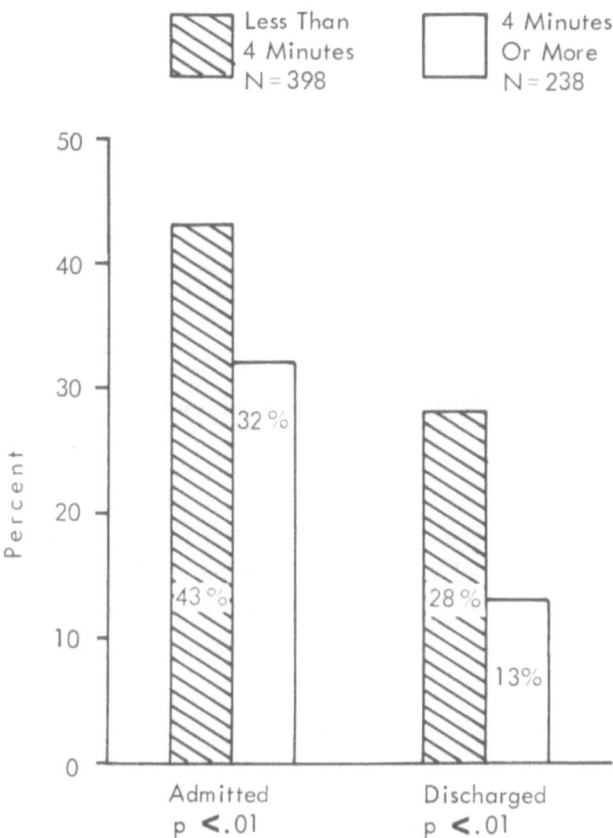

Figure 2. Time to initiation of CPR and outcome for cardiac arrests due to heart disease in King County, Washington.

discharged compared to 9% of patients if this type of care is provided in more than 14 min (Figure 3).

Many programs have been set up to train lay citizens in cardiopulmonary resuscitation and thus provide the opportunity for CPR to be initiated rapidly at the scene. Seattle has pioneered the concept of citizen CPR training and a special program was established which has trained approximately 30% of the population in cardiopulmonary resuscitation [32].

Clearly, the life-saving benefit of paramedic programs is due to the fact that they can provide definitive care directly at the scene. If they are to be effective, they must provide this care within approximately 10 min of the time from dispatch. Furthermore, for maximum effectiveness the patient must have CPR initiated at the scene within 4 min of the time from collapse. The relationship of survival to rapid provision of CPR and definitive care clearly demonstrate that the system itself is responsible for saving patients from cardiac arrest. To merely place many units on the street providing paramedic level care would be a naive attempt at saving lives.

162

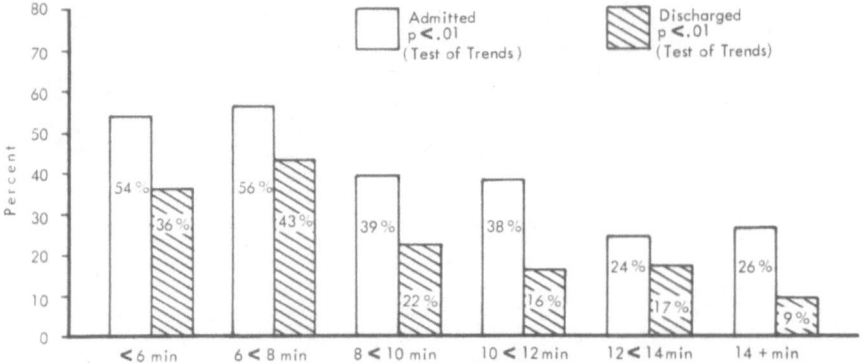

Figure 3. Time from collapse to definitive care and outcome of cardiac arrest due to heart disease in King County, Washington.

But the integration of the system with other training programs such as citizen CPR and basic emergency medical technician care, effective public access to emergency telephone numbers, efficient communication between hospital and paramedics, and other factors are the reasons that some programs are able to achieve significant success.

3.3. Potential effectiveness

It is difficult to estimate the number of lives which could be saved if efficient paramedic services were established nationally. Paramedic programs are not present throughout all urban centers and, furthermore, the data reported above demonstrate the difficulty in drawing generalizations about effectiveness of paramedic programs. This is partly because of the methodologic inconsistencies of the numerous studies and because of the lack of consistent case definition and reporting of the data. Nonetheless, some theoretical assumptions may be possible. It is estimated in the United States that half of the 700 000 deaths due to coronary artery disease occur suddenly out of the hospital. Approximately two-thirds of these patients have ventricular fibrillation as the cardiac rhythm responsible for collapse. Since the best survival rates for out of hospital ventricular fibrillation are approximately 35%, then theoretically 82 000 lives per year could be saved. Of course, these are only predictions and represent a hypothetical upper limit.

4. UNANSWERED QUESTIONS

As demonstrated above, the extent of effectiveness of paramedic programs is only partially quantified. Clearly, paramedics can save cardiac arrest patients. It is not clear, however, if there is any benefit for patients with myocardial infarction.

Furthermore, studies have not yet been done measuring the effectiveness, if any, of paramedic programs for other medical emergencies or for traumatic emergencies.

5. SUMMARY

Radical changes have occurred in the delivery of out-of-hospital emergency care. Beginning in the late 1960's, hundreds of thousands of emergency medical technicians were trained to provide a basic standard of care for out-of-hospital emergencies. While the early emphasis was on the management of trauma, the development of paramedic programs in the 1970's added an emphasis for the management of cardiac arrest patients. Numerous case series and one control study demonstrate the effectiveness of paramedic programs in dealing with cardiac arrest emergencies. Some reasons for the effectiveness have been shown and these primarily have to do with fate and system factors. The benefit of paramedic programs for other medical or traumatic emergencies has not been demonstrated.

ACKNOWLEDGEMENTS

We wish to thank the Project Restart staff, including Linda Becker, Sheri Shaeffer, Rob Galbraith, Barbara Blake and Barbara Baldwin, who assisted in collecting data of the King County, Wash. and analyzing these. Special thanks are due the King County Emergency Medical Services Division and its manager, Judith Pierce, for their ongoing hospitality and support. This work was supported in part by Grant Number HS 02456, National Center for Health Services Research, Health Resources Administration.

REFERENCES

1. Sadler AN, Sadler BL, Webb SB, Jr: Emergency Medical Care: The Neglected Public Service. Cambridge, MA: Ballinger, 1977.
2. National Academy of Sciences, National Research Council, Division of Medical Sciences Report: Accidental Death and Disability: the Neglected Disease of Modern Society. Washington, D.C., 1966.
3. Emergency Care and Transportation for the Sick and Injured; 2nd ed., American Academy of Orthopaedic Surgeons, 1971.
4. Pantridge JF, Geddes JS: Cardiac arrest after myocardial infarction. Lancet 1:807–808, 1966.
5. Pantridge JF, Geddes JS: A mobile intensive care unit in the management of myocardial infarction. Lancet 2:271–273, 1967.
6. Grace WJ, Chadbourne JA: The mobile coronary care unit. Dis Chest 55:452–455, 1969.
7. Romano TL, Eisenberg S, Fernandez-Caballero C, Cayten CG: Paramedic service: Nationwide distribution and management structure. JACEP 7:99–102, 1978.
8. National training course, Emergency Medical Technician Paramedic, U.S. Department of Transportation, National Highway Traffic Safety Administration, 1977.

9. Pozen MW, Fried DD, Smith S, Lindsay L, Voight GG: Studies of ambulance patients with ischemic heart disease: I. The outcome of pre-hospital life-threatening arrhythmias in patients receiving electrocardiographic telemetry therapeutic interventions. Am J Public Health 67:527–531, 1977.

10. Pozen MW, Fried DD, Voight GG: Studies of ambulance patients with ischemic heart disease: II. Selection of patients for ambulance telemetry. Am J Public Health 67:532–535, 1977.

11. Crampton RS, Aldrich RF, Gascho JA, Miles JR, Stillerman R: Reduction of prehospital, ambulance and community coronary death rates by the community wide emergency cardiac care system. Am J Med 58:151–165, 1975.

12. Crampton RS, Aldrich RF, Stillerman R, Gascho JA, Miles, JR: Influence of pre-hospital emergency cardiac care upon mortality from coronary artery disease. Para-Med J, Winter, 1974.

13. Lauterbach SA, Spadafora M, Levy R: Evaluation of cardiac arrests managed by paramedics. JACEP 7:355–357, 1978.

14. Lewis RP, Stang JM, Fulkerson PK, et al: Effectiveness of advanced paramedics in a mobile coronary care system. JAMA 241:1902–1904, 1979.

15. Iseri LT, Siner EI, Humphrey SB, Mann S: Prehospital cardiac arrest after arrival of the paramedic unit. JACEP 6:530–535, 1977.

16. Eisenberg MS, Bergner L, Hallstrom A: Paramedic programs and out-of-hospital cardiac arrest: I. Factors associated with successful resuscitations. Am J Public Health 69:30–38, 1979.

17. Eisenberg MS, Bergner L, Hallstrom A: Paramedic programs and out-of-hospital cardiac arrest: II. Impact on community mortality. Am J Public Health 69:39–42, 1979.

18. Bergner L, Eisenberg MS, Hallstrom A, Becker L: Evaluation of Paramedic Services for Cardiac Arrest. Unpublished Final Report for Grant Number HS02456. Report submitted to the National Center for Health Services Research, Department of Health and Human Services, Washington D.C., 1980.

19. Carveth SW, Olson D, Bechtel J: Emergency medical care system: Lincoln (Neb) mobile heart team. Arch Surg 108:528–530, 1974.

20. Graf WS, Polin SS, Paegel BL: A community program for emergency cardiac care. JAMA 226: 156–160, 1973.

21. Liberthson RR, Nagel EL, Hirschman JC, Nussenfeld SR: Prehospital ventricular defibrillation: Prognosis and follow-up course. N Engl J Med 291:317–321, 1974.

22. Nagel EL, Liberthson RR, Hirschman JC, Nussenfeld SR: Emergency care. Circulation 51 and 52 (Suppl 3):216–218, 1975.

23. Rockswold G, Sharma B, Ruiz E, et al: Follow-up of 514 consecutive patients with cardiopulmonary arrest outside the hospital. JACEP 8:216–220, 1979.

24. Rose LB: The Oregon coronary ambulance project: an experiment. Heart and Lung 3:753–755, 1974.

25. Cobb LA, Baum RS, Alvarez H, Schaffer WA: Resuscitation from out-of-hospital ventricular fibrillation: 4 year follow-up. Circulation 51 and 52 (Suppl 3):223–228, 1975.

26. Cobb LA, Werner JA, Trobaugh GB: Sudden cardiac death: I. A decade's experience with out-of-hospital resuscitation. Mod Concepts Cardiovasc Dis XLIX:31–36, 1980.

27. Cobb LA, Werner JA, Trobaugh GB: Sudden cardiac death. II. Outcome of resuscitation, management, and future directions. Mod Concepts Cardiovasc Dis XLIX:37–42, 1980.

28. Eliastam M, Duralde T, Martinez S et al.: Cardiac arrest in the emergency medical service system: guidelines for resuscitation. JACEP 6:525–529, 1977.

29. Amey BD, Harrison EE, Staub EJ: Sudden cardiac death: A retrospective and prospective study. JACEP 5:429–433, 1976.

30. Diamond JN, Schofferman J, Elliott JW: Factors in successful resuscitation by paramedics. JACEP 6:42–46, 1977.

31. Sherman MA: Mobile intensive care units: An evaluation of effectiveness. JAMA 241:1899–1901, 1979.

32. Cobb LA, Hallstrom AP, Thompson RG et al.: Community cardiopulmonary resuscitation. Ann Rev Med 31:453–462, 1980.

10. PATHOPHYSIOLOGY, CLINICAL COURSE, AND MANAGEMENT OF PREHOSPITAL VENTRICULAR FIBRILLATION AND SUDDEN CARDIAC DEATH

RICHARD R. LIBERTHSON, EUGENE L. NAGEL, and
JEREMY N. RUSKIN

This chapter is divided into four sections, each dealing with a different aspect of the problem of prehospital ventricular fibrillation and sudden cardiac death as encountered by the authors during the past decade. It includes the clinical and pathophysiologic characterization of this population, the hospital and follow-up course of resuscitated patients, and our present approach to the long-term management of resuscitated survivors. This work was published in greater detail during the past decade [1–3] and is presented here in abbreviated form. We are indebted to our many co-workers who made these studies possible.[1]

1. CHARACTERIZATION OF THE PREHOSPITAL SUDDEN CARDIAC DEATH POPULATION

In the city of Miami 300 witnessed victims of prehospital sudden cardiac death were identified between 1970 and 1973 [1] (Table 1). All had been functioning normally in their usual environment prior to arrest. All were monitored by fire rescue squads during attempted resuscitation, and all had postmortem verification of the absence of noncardiac causes for sudden death. In all, a detailed remote, recent and acute medical history was obtained by trained interviewers using detailed questionaires[2]. As detailed in Table 1, this was predominantly a male and a Caucasian population – 84 and 86%, respectively. A prior history of cardiovascular disease was present in many of them including remote myocardial infarction (36%), angina pectoris (49%), and hypertension (34%).

During the four weeks preceding cardiac arrest, new or changing symptoms of chest pain and/or dyspnea were reported in 29%, with half of this percentage starting within one week. Twenty-nine percent had consulted a physician within one month of their cardiac arrest, often because of new or changing symptoms. On the day of cardiac arrest, 28% reported new chest pain and/or dyspnea which preceded the arrest by more than 30 min. However, these did not alter their activity or prompt

---

[1] Drs. Jim C. Hirschman, Sidney R. Nussenfeld, Brian D. Blackbourne, Joseph H. Davis, Hasan Garan, and John P. DiMarco.
[2] Copies available from the Myocardial Infarction Branch of the National Heart, Blood, and Lung Institute, Bethesda, MA, U.S.A.

Adgey, AAJ (ed): Acute phase of ischemic heart disease and myocardial infarction.
© *1982, Martinus Nijhoff, The Hague, Boston, London. ISBN-13: 978-94-009-7581-1*

166

them to seek medical help. In 24%, only very acute symptoms of chest pain or dyspnea were present which preceded arrest by less than 30 min (mean 13 min). Approximately one-half of the victims collapsed instantaneously.

Forty-three percent of arrests occurred at home and 13% while at work. Activity immediately preceding the arrest was strenuous or psychologically stressful in 20%, and mild or moderate in the remainder.

2. PATHOLOGIC CHARACTERIZATION OF PREHOSPITAL SUDDEN CARDIAC DEATH

Between 1970 and 1973, 220 of the victims of witnessed, monitored sudden cardiac death characterized in Table 1 underwent detailed postmortem evaluation in the

Table 1. Characterization of monitored sudden cardiac death victims (N = 300)

Male/mean age	84% / 55 years
Female/mean age	16% / 59 years
Negro	14%
Caucasian	86%
Blue collar	42%
White collar	40%
Professional	5%
Retired	13%
History of old myocardial infarction	36%
History of angina pectoris or chest pain	49%
History of hypertension	34%
More than 10 cigarettes a day	63%
History of diabetes mellitus	11%
Over-normal height-weight index (male)	45%
Over-normal height-weight index (female)	60%
New or changing symptoms within 4 weeks	29%
Physician visits within 4 weeks	29%
Visits for new symptoms	16%
Warning symptoms on day of acute event	28%
Mean interval	3.6. h
Acute terminal symptoms only	24%
Mean interval	13 min
Sudden collapse without prior symptoms	49%
Location of acute event	
Home	43%
Work	13%
Public place	44%
Activity immediately preceding acute event	
Rest or sleep	20%
Mild or moderate	60%
Strenuous or stressful	20%

Table 2. Pathologic characterization of sudden cardiac death victims (N = 220)

Average heart weight		
Male	190 cases	460 g
Female	30 cases	374 g
Coronary pattern		
Dominant right	86%	
Dominant left	10%	
Balanced	4%	
No coronary stenosis	6%	
Stenosis over 75%	94%	
One vessel		14%
Two vessel		26%
Three or four vessel		60%
Old myocardial infarction	44%	
Anterior wall		20%
Anterior and inferior wall		29%
Inferior wall		51%
Acute coronary occlusion	58%	
Single vessel		84%
Multiple vessels		16%
Ruptured plaque		56%
Thrombosis		32%
Intramural hemorrhage		10%
Embolus		2%
Acute myocardial infarction	27%	
Anterior wall		22%
Anterior and inferior wall		12%
Inferior wall		66%
Very fresh (< 1 day)		17%
Fresh (1–3 days)		39%
Recent (3–7 days)		17%
Organizing (1 week)		27%

Medical Examiner's Office of the City of Miami using specially prepared study protocols[3] [1] (Table 2). Strict adherence to methodology and to definitions as outlined below was maintained. Studies were performed by Drs. Joseph Davis and Brian Blackbourne.

2.1. Pathology definitions

The major coronary arteries and their branches were dissected free, fixed in formaldehyde, decalcified, and cut in cross-sections at 1 mm intervals. Acute lesions and severely stenotic segments were embedded in paraffin and alternate sections were stained with hematoxylin and eosin (H and E) and, in some cases, Weigert Van

[3] See note 2.

Gieson stains. The myocardium was sectioned from apex to base at 0.5 cm intervals. All overt lesions as well as routine sections from the mid-septum and mid-anterior, lateral, and inferior walls were fixed in formaldehyde, embedded, stained with H and E, and studied under a light microscope. Acute coronary artery lesions were classified as thrombosis, plaque rupture, or intramural hemorrhage according to the following definitions:

– Thrombosis was defined as 'fresh' when the red blood cell, platelet, and fibrin mass were loosely attached to the intimal lining but showed no organization or 'organizing' when the thrombus was adherent to the intima and when there was fibroblast proliferation.

– Plaque Rupture was defined as a disruption of the intimal wall overlying the plaque with extrusion of plaque substance into the coronary lumen. Included in this group were cases in which rupture was complicated by overlying thrombus or dissecting intramural hemorrhage.

– Intramural Hemorrhage was defined as hemorrhage into a plague with persistence of an intact intimal lining.

– Acute Myocardial Infarction was defined as 'very fresh' when there was increased eosinophils, blurred cross-striations, and hyalinization and vacuolization of myocardial fibers but nuclear details were still present (less than one day old); 'fresh' when the above changes were accompanied by loss of cellular detail and early polymorphonuclear granulocyte infiltration (one to three days old); 'recent' when necrosis was well delineated and associated with heavy polymorphonuclear granulocyte infiltration and early absorption of necrotic debris (three to seven days old); and 'organizing' when capillary and fibroblast proliferation were present (one to two weeks old).

– Severe Chronic Stenosis was defined as narrowing of more than 75% of the coronary lumen area estimated from standard planimetered templates.[4] Acute and chronic coronary artery lesions located in the first 3 cm of the involved vessel were considered proximal. Old myocardial infarction was defined as a fibrous scar 1 cm or more in diameter. These were either solid or patchy.

2.2. Pathology findings

Acute changes

Acute myocardial infarction was detected in 59 autopsied subjects (27%) (Table 2). It involved the anterior wall in 22%, the inferior wall in 66%, and both anterior and inferior walls in 12% of the subjects. In only 10 subjects with acute myocardial infarction (17%) these changes were less than one day old, and in the remainder they exceeded 24 hours in age. Five patients had a ruptured ventricular wall and one had a ruptured papillary muscle.

Acute coronary lesions were present in 128 victims (58%). In 108, a single cor-

---

[4] See note 2.

Table 3. Cardiac rhythm present on arrival of rescue workers (N = 426)

Ventricular fibrillation	72%
Idioventricular rhythm	8%
Asystole	8%
Junctional rhythm	7%
Sinus bradycardia	2%
Atrio-ventricular block	2%
Ventricular tachycardia	1%

onary artery was involved, and in 20 subjects more than one vessel had acute changes. Acute coronary lesions involved the right coronary artery in 48% of victims, the LAD in 33%, the left main in 3%, and left circumflex in 16%. Acute coronary lesions were most often ruptured plaques, viz. 72 subjects (56% of those with acute coronary changes). Thrombosis without discernible intimal rupture was found in 42 subjects, i.e. 32% of those with acute coronary lesions and 19% of all sudden cardiac deaths (SCD's) autopsied and these were fresh or recent in 32 and organizing in 10. Intramural hemorrhage was found in 14 subjects (10%). Acute coronary lesions occurred at the site of severe old stenosis in all but four subjects.

In 81 subjects (37%) no acute vascular or myocardial lesion was found. Acute coronary or myocardial changes in patients with symptoms prior to death were slightly different from those with no known symptoms. In those with preceding symptoms, 33% had detectable acute infarction, 66% had acute coronary lesions, and 25% had neither acute myocardial nor vascular changes. In those with no reported prior symptoms, 16% had detectable acute infarctions, 48% had acute coronary lesions, and 51% had no acute changes. Preceding symptoms did not vary with different types of acute coronary lesions nor did the degree of activity immediately prior to collapse.

Chronic changes

Chronic coronary artery stenosis of more than 75% of the lumen area was present in 207 subjects (94%). In 13 subjects (6%), no severe chronic stenosis was present, and of these, 1 had myocarditis, 4 had cardiomyopathy, 3 had coronary emboli, 1 had coronary arteritis, and 4 had severe valvular heart disease.

In 29 subjects (14%), only one major vessel was stenosed, 2 of them having total old occlusion. In these subjects, the left anterior descending (LAD) coronary artery was involved in 19, the left main in 2, the right in 6, and the left circumflex in 2. These lesions were proximal in 23 subjects (19 LAD and 4 right). Thus, in the subgroup of sudden death victims who had only a single abnormal coronary artery, 21 of 29 subjects (72%) had a proximal lesion of the artery supplying the major circulation for the anterior wall of the left ventricle. Seventeen of these victims (59%) had a demonstrable acute occlusion, and five (17%) also had histologic changes of acute infarction. Hearts with stenosis of a single vessel had an average weight of 371 g.

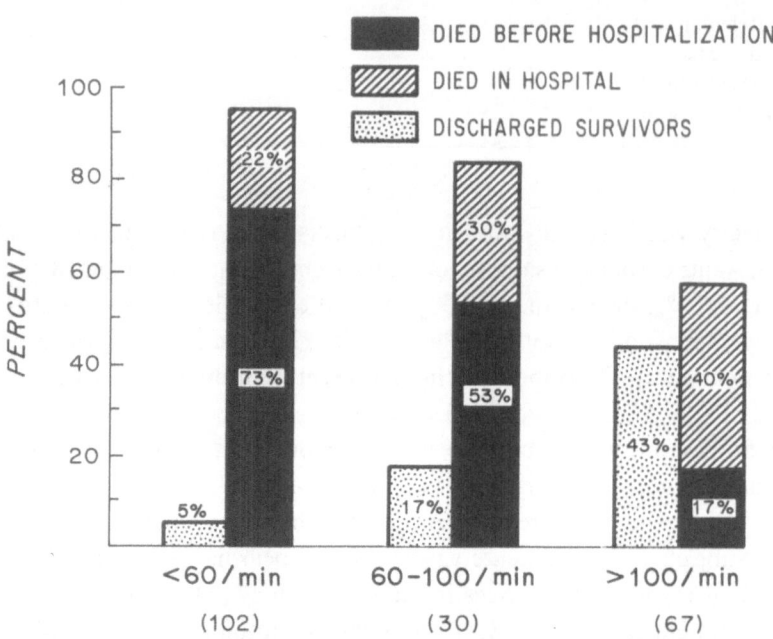

Figure 1. Prognostic implications of initial post-defibrillation heart rate. (Reprinted by permission of the N Engl J Med 291:317–321, 1974.)

In 53 subjects (26%), two major arteries had severe old stenosis with total occlusion in 14. Acute coronary lesions were found in 28 of them (53%) and acute infarction in 11 (21%). These heart weights averaged 429 g.

In 125 subjects (60%), severe old stenosis involved three or four vessels with total occlusion in 56. Acute coronary lesions were found in 82 in this group (65%) and acute infarction in 43 (34%). The weight of these hearts averaged 459 g.

An old infarction was present in 97 subjects (44%), and these scars were distributed equally between the anterior and inferior walls.

3. CLINICAL OBSERVATIONS AND COURSE OF RESUSCITATED PREHOSPITAL VENTRICULAR FIBRILLATION VICTIMS

Between 1970 and 1973, 426 monitored prehospital sudden unexpected cardiac arrest victims in the City of Miami were reviewed [1, 2]. The cardiac rhythms present in these subjects on arrival of fire rescue, which averaged 3 min from time of summons in 84% of the cases and which averaged less than 15 min of observed collapse in

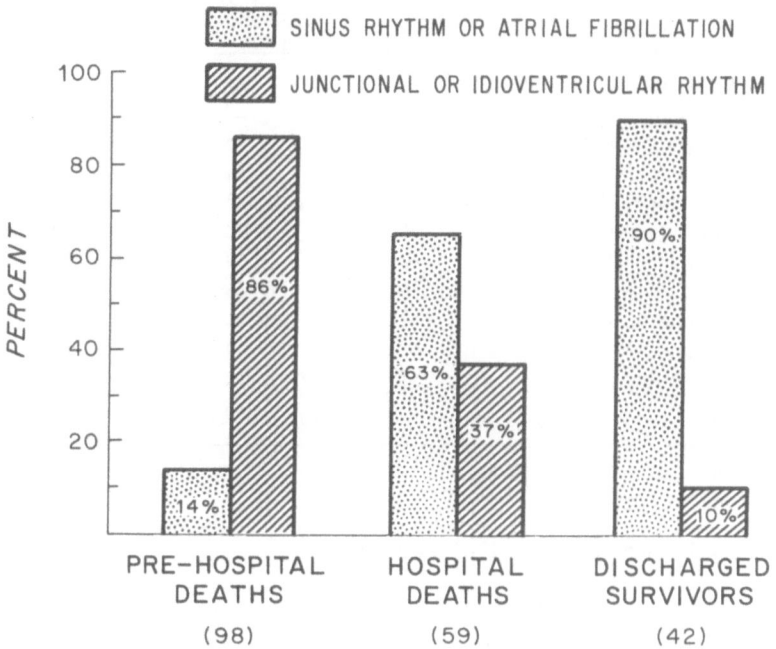

PROGNOSTIC IMPLICATIONS OF
INITIAL POST–DEFIBRILLATION CARDIAC RHYTHM

Figure 2. Prognostic implications of initial post-defibrillation cardiac rhythm. (Reprinted by permission of the N Engl J Med 291:317–321, 1974.)

90%, are detailed in Table 3. Noteworthy is the presence of ventricular fibrillation in nearly three-quarters of these victims.

3.1. Prehospital course of monitored cardiac arrests

The initial post-defibrillation heart rate recorded within one minute of defibrillation in relation to the subjects' clinical outcome is shown in Figure 1. Of the 199 successful defibrillations, 102 subjects had initial post-defibrillation heart rates of less than 60 per min, 30 had rates between 60 and 100 per min, and 67 had heart rates of more than 100 per min. Of those with rates below 60 per min, 5% survived through discharge, 22% died in the hospital, and 73% died before hospitalization. Of those with heart rates between 60 and 100 per min, 17% survived through discharge, 30% died in the hospital, and 53% died before admission. Of those with initial post-defibrillation heart rates greater than 100 per min, 43% survived through discharge, 40% died in the hospital, and 17% died before hospitalization.[5] The estimated mean

[5] Survival when heart rates greater than 100 per minute were compared to rates less than 60 per minute was statistically significant at $p < 0.001$, as was survival with atrial fibrillation or sinus rhythm as compared to idioventricular or junctional rhythms (chi-square method).

172

Table 4. Hospital follow-up data on surviving patients who had defibrillation (N = 101)

	Hospital deaths %	Discharged survivors %	Totals %
Acute myocardial infarction	37	31	35
Ischemia without infarction	34	29	32
No acute electrocardiographic change	10	26	17
Complete left-bundle-branch block[a]	19	14	17
Complete right-bundle-branch block	24	7	17
Repeat ventricular fibrillation	50	24	40
Congestive heart failure	69	53	63
Cardiogenic shock	39	5	25
Severe pulmonary complications[b]	41	44	42
Severe neurologic deficit	95	12	61
Partial neurologic deficit	5	28	15
No neurologic deficit	—	60	25

[a] Possibly masking an acute myocardial change.
[b] Aspiration pneumonia or flail chest.

(Reprinted, by permission of N Engl J Med 291:317–321, 1974).

interval from witnessed collapse until defibrillation was 10 min in those with initial post-defibrillation heart rates greater than 100 per min and 16 min in those with rates less than 60 per min.

The initial post-defibrillation cardiac rhythm in these subjects is shown in Figure 2. Idioventricular or junctional rhythms were present in 86% of prehospital deaths, 37% of hospital deaths, and 10% of discharged survivors; atrial fibrillation or sinus rhythm was present in 14% of prehospital deaths, 63% of hospital deaths, and 90% of discharged survivors.

3.2. Hospital course of successfully resuscitated patients

Between 1970 and 1973, 101 resuscitated survivors of prehospital ventricular fibrillation were hospitalized primarily at the Jackson Memorial Hospital in the City of Miami [2] (Table 4). Of those hospitalized, 42 survived through discharge, and 59 died in the hospital. Electrocardiographic evidence of acute myocardial infarction was present in 35% of hospitalized patients, and myocardial ischemia alone in 32%. Both were equally frequent in survivors and in those who died. Complete left bundle branch block was present in 17% and precluded electrocardiographic diagnosis of acute myocardial change. In 17% of patients – 10% of those who died in the hospital and 26% of discharged survivors – no acute myocardial changes evolved on serial

Table 5. Localization of acute electrocardiographic myocardial changes in defibrillated survivors (N = 58)

	Patients	
	No.	%
Acute myocardial infarction	31	
Anterior wall	16	52%
Anterior and inferior wall	4	13%
Inferior wall	11	35%
Ischemia without infarction	27	
Anterior wall	19	70%
Anterior and inferior wall	5	19%
Inferior wall	3	11%

electrocardiograms.[6] Seven patients had severe valvular heart disease (4 of whom had acute myocardial changes as well).

The ECG diagnosis of myocardial change in defibrillated survivors of 'would-be SCD's' provided a more accurate estimate of the incidence and anatomic location of acute myocardial changes in this population than did standard histologic study of similar victims at postmortem examination. This is owing to the fact that defibrillation reverses the otherwise terminal course of ventricular fibrillation and permits detection of early myocardial changes, notably ischemia, that would otherwise be unrecognized histologically if immediate death occurred. In resuscitated patients, we observed that ECG evidence for acute myocardial change, whether infarction or ischemia, occurred in 67% of patients (Table 4) in contrast to only 27% who had acute histologic myocardial changes at postmortem (Table 2). While it is possible that in some resuscitated patients acute myocardial changes evolved secondary to arrest and resuscitation, it is equally possible that this estimate is accurate, as others have observed a similar incidence of acute myocardial changes in autopsied sudden cardiac deaths using highly sensitive histochemical pathological techniques or myocardial sodium-potassium ratios for detecting very early myocardial changes.

Of note, there is a marked disparity between the anatomic location of ischemia seen in defibrillated survivors (Table 5) and that of acute histologic myocardial infarction in autopsied sudden death victims (Table 2) which provides possible insight into the initiation of ventricular fibrillation in these victims. As shown in Table 5, in defibrillated survivors who have ECG ischemic changes, the anterior wall alone was involved in 70%, the inferior wall alone in 11%, and both walls in 19%. In

---

[6] Serum enzyme data were not used for the diagnosis of acute myocardial change because all patients were defibrillated. These enzymes, however, were evaluated in 87 patients and were elevated in 83. Myocardial specific isoenzyme assessment was not available at the time of this study nor was thallium imaging.

contrast to these ischemic changes, those with histologic changes of transmural myocardial infarction (Table 2), in only 22% the anterior wall alone was involved, in 66% the inferior wall was involved, and in 12% both walls were involved. This disparity suggests that anterior wall lesions precipitate ventricular fibrillation too rapidly to allow histologic detection with the aid of standard techniques that are useful for lesions only older than 8 h. Thus, only if defibrillation permits survival do the greater number of acute myocardial changes and the anterior wall predominance of these lesions as observed in resuscitated survivors become evident. This possible relationship between anterior wall lesions and rapid ventricular fibrillation highlights the need for intensive antiarrhythmic prophylaxis in patients with extensive compromise of the anterior wall perfusion, particularly when associated with new or changing symptoms.

Ventricular fibrillation recurred after admission in 40% of patients (83% on the first hospital day) and was twice as frequent among patients who died in the hospital than among discharged survivors (Table 4). Ventricular tachycardia in the absence of ventricular fibrillation occurred in 17% of patients (all on the first hospital day) and frequent premature ventricular contractions in the absence of either ventricular fibrillation or ventricular tachycardia were noted in 26%. Ventricular irritability in all patients was managed according to standard coronary care unit practice during the study period. In 17% of patients – 9 who died in the hospital and 9 discharged survivors – no significant ventricular irritability was detected throughout the hospital course. Of the latter patients, three quarters had either rapid atrial fibrillation or sinus tachycardia.

Moderate or severe congestive heart failure was present in 63% of patients and cardiogenic shock in 25% (Table 4). Only two of the latter were discharged alive. Serious pulmonary complications were present in 42 patients (42%), including aspiration pneumonia in 33 patients and flail chest in 23, and they were equally frequent among survivors and those who died. The presence of pulmonary complications prolonged hospital stay, but did not affect mortality.

In four cases (all hospital deaths) complete atrioventricular block occurred. Complete right bundle branch block was present in 17% of patients (24% of those who died in the hospital and 7% of survivors). Bifascicular block was present in 15 patients which, in 5 patients, was known to have preceded cardiac arrest. In 5 patients bifascicular block was known to be acute, and in 5 it was of unknown duration.

Death in the hospital occurred on the first day of admission in 41%, from one day to one week in 34%, and from one week to one month in 25%. Of those who survived through discharge, 60% returned to their pre-arrest way of life, 28% returned home but had partial neurologic impairment, and 12% had severe deficit which required institutional care (Table 4).

3.3. Post-discharge course of survivors

Twenty-two of the 42 survivors were alive at a mean follow-up of 16.8 months and a median of 13 months, and 20 had died with a mean and median survival of 8.3 months and 6 months, respectively. Sudden death following discharge occurred in 12 patients (28 percent). In five of these deaths, ventricular fibrillation was again monitored by rescue workers. Two patients survived two episodes of prehospital ventricular fibrillation. Of the 12 who died suddenly after discharge, 4 had acute myocardial infarction during the hospital course (all involving the anterior wall), 4 had only ischemia (all involving the anterior wall), 1 had left bundle branch block, and 3 had no demonstrable myocardial changes.

In 29 patients, one or more antiarrhythmic agents were prescribed after discharge. These drugs were prescribed according to standard practice in the community during the study period and varied considerably among different physicians and patients. They included quinidine in 14, procainamide in 13, propranolol in 3, and diphenylhydantoin in 2 patients. In 13 patients, no antiarrhythmics were prescribed after discharge, generally because significant dysrhythmia was not observed in the hospital. Of the 29 patients discharged on antiarrhythmic agents, 14 were alive and 15 died (10 of whom suddenly) at 18 months follow-up, and of the 13 patients discharged with no antiarrhythmic agents, 8 were living, and 5 had died (two of whom suddenly). During the study period aortocoronary artery bypass surgery was performed in 6 patients after their episode of ventricular fibrillation. Of these, 4 were alive and 2 died (one of whom suddenly) at 18 months follow-up.

4. PRESENT CLINICAL MANAGEMENT OF THE DISCHARGED SURVIVOR OF VENTRICULAR FIBRILLATION

The very high mortality secondary to recurrent ventricular fibrillation on follow-up of discharged survivors of prehospital ventricular fibrillation (in the absence of acute myocardial infarction) is now well known and approximates 30% [2]. This incidence has changed little in spite of intensive 'standard' antiarrhythmic management or coronary artery bypass grafting. In an attempt to reduce the high rate of recurrent ventricular fibrillation, recent studies using intensive electrophysiologic investigation of these patients and tailored antiarrhythmic drug protocols have been undertaken. This work was performed in conjunction with Drs. Hasan Garan and John DiMarco at the Massachusetts General Hospital in the laboratory directed by Dr. Jeremy Ruskin [3].

Between 1978 and 1981, 61 survivors of prehospital cardiac arrest unassociated with acute myocardial infarction were studied at the Massachusetts General Hospital, Boston, Mass. At the time of resuscitation, ventricular fibrillation was present in 52 patients and ventricular tachycardia in 9 patients.

The patient population included 47 men and 14 women ranging in age from 19 to 74 years (mean 56 years). Atherosclerotic coronary artery disease was present in 46 patients, valvular heart disease in 6 patients, and primary myocardial disease in 5 patients. In 4 patients, no evidence of structural heart disease was detected by invasive or noninvasive study. Initial electrophysiologic studies were performed an average of 3 weeks after resuscitation from cardiac arrest. Following resuscitation, 8 patients received 3-vessel aortocoronary saphenous vein bypass grafts because of either advanced disease of the left main coronary artery or severe proximal 3-vessel coronary artery disease. Two additional patients underwent left ventricular aneurysmectomy. In 9 of these 10 surgical patients, electrophysiologic studies were performed both before and 2 weeks after cardiac surgery; in 1 patient studies were deferred until after surgery because of a nearly complete left main coronary artery ostial occlusion.

4.1. Electrophysiology study methods

Patients were studied in a fasting, non-sedated state. Cardiac medications taken at the time of cardiac arrest were discontinued at least 48 h before the initial electrophysiologic study in all but 2 patients. Digitalis therapy was continued for the control of congestive heart failure in 15 patients. Electrode catheters were inserted percutaneously via femoral or antecubital veins and positioned under fluoroscopic guidance at multiple intracardiac sites. Cardiac stimulation was performed with a programmable constant-current stimulator (Medtronic 5325) that delivered rectangular pulses of 2 ms duration at twice the diastolic threshold. In all but 3 patients with inducible arrhythmias, induction occurred with right ventricular apical stimulation. In 3 patients, ventricular arrhythmias were initiated only with stimulation of the right ventricular outflow tract. The following stimulation protocol was used: incremental atrial pacing (100–300 beats per min), premature atrial stimulation during atrial pacing, incremental ventricular pacing (60–150 beats per min), premature right ventricular stimulation with single and double extrastimuli during ventricular pacing, and brief bursts (2–5 beats) of rapid ventricular pacing at rates of 150–280 beats per min. If sustained ventricular tachycardia was initiated, bursts of rapid ventricular pacing at rates of 150–300 beats per min were applied for 5–20 beats to interrupt the arrhythmia. If an induced arrhythmia caused loss of consciousness or compromised perfusion, asynchronous external electrical countershock was performed immediately.
- Sustained Ventricular Tachycardia was defined as tachycardia that persisted for at least 100 beats and required pacing or external countershock for termination.
- Nonsustained Ventricular Tachycardia was defined as tachycardia that persisted for at least five beats and reverted spontaneously within 100 beats to normal sinus rhythm.
- Repetitive Responses observed in two patients were defined as three or more beats of ventricular origin that occurred reproducibly in response to programmed stimulation.

Among the 61 patients, inducible ventricular arrhythmias occurred in 50 of them (82%) during programmed cardiac stimulation. In 4 patients, ventricular tachycardia could be initiated only during therapy with the same antiarrhythmic drug that had been present at the time of cardiac arrest; tachycardia could not be initiated in these patients in the absence of antiarrhythmic drugs. In 43 of 50 patients with inducible ventricular arrhythmias, serial drug tests were performed in an attempt to define an antiarrhythmic drug regimen that would ensure that the ventricular arrhythmia observed at the time of the initial study could no longer be initiated by programmed ventricular stimulation. We serially tested each of a number of standard antiarrhythmic drug regimens that were selected on the basis of patient tolerance, ease of administration, and drug history. After the patient had received a loading dose of each drug and oral maintenance therapy for at least 48 h, electrophysiologic testing was repeated. Plasma concentrations of these drugs were determined at the time of testing. The drugs were administered in standard therapeutic doses and included, quinidine sulfate, procainamide, disopyramide, phenytoin, and propranolol. Disopyramide and propranolol were not tested in any patient with severe left ventricular dysfunction.

If the initiation of ventricular arrhythmias could not be prevented with currently approved antiarrhythmic drugs, electrophysiologic testing was carried out with one or more investigational drugs including mexiletine, tocainide, amiodarone, and aprindine. Because rapid methods to determine plasma concentrations of these agents were not available, the dose of each drug was increased until either a therapeutic effect or a toxic side effect was observed.

The efficacy of these antiarrhythmic drugs was assessed by repeat electrophysiologic testing using an indwelling bipolar right ventricular apical electrode that was inserted via a subclavian vein and left in place throughout the testing period (2–14 days). The stimulation protocol used during serial drug testing was identical to that described above. Patients were followed at three-month intervals after a final antiarrhythmic drug regimen was selected on the basis of the results of serial electrophysiologic testing.

4.2. Electrophysiologic observations

Of the 61 survivors of out-of-hospital cardiac arrest, 50 had electrically inducible ventricular arrhythmias in response to programmed cardiac stimulation. The arrhythmias observed included sustained ventricular tachycardia in 17 patients, nonsustained ventricular tachycardia in 25, ventricular fibrillation in 6, and repetitive ventricular responses of 3–4 beats in 2 (Figure 3). Premature ventricular stimulation alone initiated ventricular arrhythmias in 29 patients; brief bursts of rapid ventricular pacing alone caused arrhythmias in 6; and both modes of ventricular stimulation were effective in 15. The mean rate of electrically induced sustained ventricular tachycardias was 210 ± 36 beats per min ranging from 165 to 300. Induced sustained ventricular tachycardia was terminated by rapid ventricular

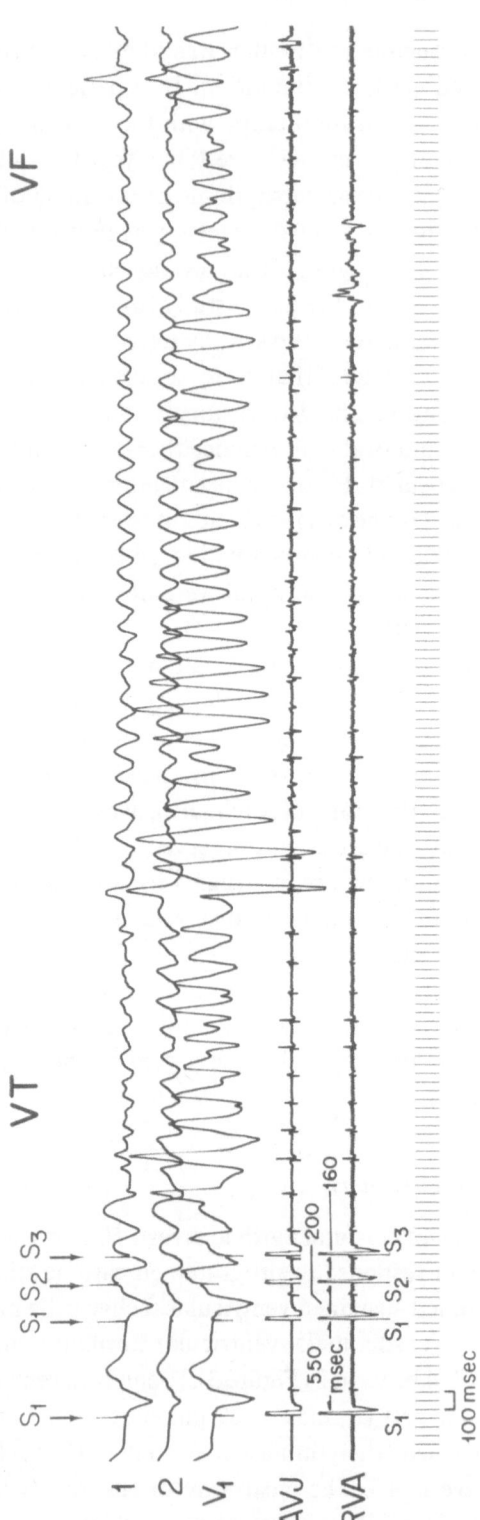

Figure 3. Initiation of ventricular fibrillation by programmed ventricular stimulation in a survivor of out-of-hospital ventricular fibrillation. Tracings from top to bottom represent surface electrocardiographic leads 1,2, and V_1, a local electrogram from the right atrioventricular junction in the region of the bundle of His (AVJ), and a local electrogram from the right ventricular apex (RVA). During right ventricular pacing at a fixed cycle length (S_1–S_1), two sequential ventricular premature depolarizations (S_2 and S_3) result in the initiation of a rapid, disorganized ventricular tachycardia (VT) that degenerates to ventricular fibrillation (VF). (Reprinted by permission of the N Engl J Med 303:607–613, 1980.)

pacing in 12 of 17 patients; external countershock was required in 5 patients who had ventricular tachycardia and in the 6 who had ventricular fibrillation (Figure 3). Sustained ventricular tachycardia was associated with presyncopal symptoms in all 17 patients before termination of the arrhythmia by rapid ventricular pacing or external countershock. The mean rate of electrically induced nonsustained ventricular tachycardia was 250 ± 34 beats per min ranging from 190 to 320. The duration of induced nonsustained ventricular tachycardia ranged from 5 to 32 beats, with a mean duration of 13 beats. If nonsustained ventricular tachycardia could be repeatedly initiated with one or more modes of ventricular stimulation, more aggressive stimulation at closer ventricular coupling intervals or faster rates of ventricular pacing was not attempted.

Eight patients had undergone aortocoronary saphenous vein bypass grafts after recovery from cardiac arrest, and two additional patients had undergone ventricular aneurysmectomy. In 6 of these 10 patients, electrophysiologic studies in the absence of drugs both before and two weeks after surgery, revealed reproducible ventricular arrhythmias. These inducible arrhythmias were fully suppressed postoperatively during serial drug testing in 4 patients while only partial suppression could be achieved in 2 patients. In 2 patients, inducible ventricular arrhythmias were observed repeatedly during preoperative electrophysiologic studies, whereas no inducible arrhythmias were observed after surgical revascularization. An additional patient, who was not studied before the operation had no electrophysiologic abnormalities when examined after surgery. The latter 3 patients were discharged without antiarrhythmic therapy. One of the 10 patients died as a result of an intraoperative complication during ventricular aneurysmectomy.

In the 10 other patients, no ventricular arrhythmias were initiated during programmed cardiac stimulation. In 7 of these 10 patients, electrophysiologic evaluation revealed no detectable abnormalities. Electrophysiologic study revealed inducible atrial flutter with 1:1 atrioventricular conduction in 1 patient and a prolonged H-V interval (75 ms) alone in 1 patient, and in the remaining patient, electrophysiologic study revealed previously unsuspected first-degree block within the bundle of His. A subsequent study documented the existence of an intermittent second degree block within this atrioventricular bundle. On the basis of these findings, the patient received a permanent ventricular pacemaker. One final patient (see above) did not undergo an initial electrophysiologic evaluation because of near-occlusion of the left main coronary artery at the ostium. Postoperative electrophysiologic study in this patient revealed no abnormalities.

4.3. Serial pharmacologic and electrophysiologic testing

Serial antiarrhythmic drug testing was carried out in conjunction with programmed cardiac stimulation in 43 of the 50 patients with inducible ventricular arrhythmias and in the one patient with inducible atrial flutter and accelerated atrioventricular conduction. A total of 151 drug trials (3.5 per patient) were carried out, each with

Table 6. Final antiarrhythmic drug regimens in 49 patients with inducible ventricular arrhythmias

Mexiletine	12
Quinidine	10
Amiodarone	4
Procainamide	1
Quinidine + Procainamide	1
Quinidine + Mexiletine	4
Quinidine + Propranolol	2
Mexiletine + Procainamide	4
Mexiletine + Disopyramide	1
Mexiletine + Propranolol	2
Amiodarone + Metoprolol	1
Disopyramide + Propranolol	1
No antiarrhythmic drugs	6

programmed cardiac stimulation. There was no mortality related to these procedures. Among the 50 patients with inducible ventricular arrhythmias, complete suppression of these arrhythmias (defined as a maximum of 2 repetitive ventricular responses during programmed ventricular stimulation) was achieved in 38 patients. In 11 patients, electrically inducible ventricular arrhythmias were present on all drug regimens tested. One patient with inducible ventricular tachycardia died as a result of noncardiac complications during cardiac surgery. Four patients in whom cardiac arrest had occurred after prolonged therapy with antiarrhythmic drugs and in whom ventricular arrhythmias could be initiated only in the presence of therapeutic plasma concentrations of the drug which had been present at the time of cardiac arrest were discharged without antiarrhythmic drugs. The inability to induce ventricular arrhythmias of any type in the absence of antiarrhythmic drugs was demonstrated in all 4 patients. The patient with inducible atrial flutter and accelerated atrioventricular conduction was treated with a combination of quinidine and propranolol, which prevented the initiation of atrial flutter and prolonged the effective refractory period of the atrioventricular node.

Of the 50 patients with inducible ventricular arrhythmias, 43 were treated with antiarrhythmic medications and 6 were discharged without antiarrhythmic agents (Table 6). Of the 43 treated patients, 27 were given a single antiarrhythmic agent and the remaining 16 required a combination therapy of two antiarrhythmic agents. Quinidine and mexiletine were the most frequently effective agents and were used alone or in combination with other drugs in 36 of the 43 patients (Table 6).

4.4. Clinical follow-up

Complete suppression of electrically inducible ventricular arrhythmias was achieved in 38 of 50 patients (Table 7). Thirty-four of these 38 patients required antiarrhythmic drug therapy for the suppression of arrhythmias, whereas 4 patients

Table 7. Electrophysiologic findings in resuscitated survivors

Total patients	61
Inducible ventricular arrhythmia	50
No inducible ventricular arrhythmia	10
Not tested until after surgical intervention	1
Follow-up (average: 20 months; range: 4–43 months)	
No inducible ventricular arrhythmia at discharge	49 (38 + 10 + 1)
Alive and well	42
Sudden deaths	2 (4%)
Other deaths	4 (CHF); 1 (CA)
Inducible ventricular arrhythmias at discharge	11
Alive and well	6
Sudden deaths	4 (36%)
Other deaths	1 (CVA)
In-hospital (intraoperative) death	1

CHF, congestive heart failure
CA, carcinoma
CVA, cerebrovascular accident

required discontinuation of long-term antiarrhythmic drug therapy in order to prevent electrical induction of the arrhythmias (see above). Among these 38 patients, there were 2 sudden deaths at a mean follow-up of 20 months (range: 4–43 months). In addition, 4 patients in this group were rehospitalized and died as a result of progressive and refractory congestive heart failure. One patient died as a result of metastatic carcinoma 10 months following hospital discharge. There have been no deaths among the 10 patients, none of whom had inducible ventricular arrhythmias at the time of initial electrophysiologic study. The one patient not studied until after surgery is alive and well.

In 11 of the 50 patients who had electrically inducible ventricular arrhythmias, complete suppression could not be achieved with any drug regimen tested. All 11 patients were maintained on regimens that decelerated or abbreviated the induced arrhythmia or that rendered initiation of the arrhythmias by programmed ventricular stimulation more difficult. Among these 11 patients, there were 5 deaths (one in the hospital) during the follow-up period, 4 of which occurred suddenly as a result of recurrent ventricular arrhythmias. One patient died as a result of a cerebrovascular accident 11 months after hospital discharge.

5. SUMMARY

Over the past decade our knowledge of the problem of prehospital sudden cardiac death has been greatly advanced. Our studies in the city of Miami have confirmed the epidemiology of this problem. The clinical profile of these victims has been

182

identified. In most, there are coronary disease risk factors and in many, acute or recent symptoms. The detailed acute and chronic pathology associated with these deaths has been clarified. In most there is severe chronic coronary and myocardial disease and in many there is an acute coronary and a myocardial lesion. In the large majority the terminal rhythm is ventricular fibrillation. The efficacy of rapid-response trained rescue squads in resuscitating these victims has been established. The hospital course of these resuscitated patients has been described. Finally, the value of intensive cardiac electrophysiologic study and tailored antiarrhythmic therapy has been demonstrated, and a dramatic decrease in the recurrence rate of post-defibrillation cardiac arrest is now possible.

REFERENCES

1. Liberthson RR, Nagel EL, Hirschman JC, Nussenfeld SR, Blackbourne BD, Davis JH: Pathophysiologic observations in prehospital ventricular fibrillation and sudden cardiac death. Circulation 49:790–798, 1974.
2. Liberthson RR, Nagel EL, Hirschman JC, Nussenfeld SR: Prehospital ventricular defibrillation: prognosis and follow-up course. N Engl J Med 291:317–321, 1974.
3. Ruskin JN, DiMarco JP, Garan H: Out-of-hospital cardiac arrest: electrophysiologic observations and selection of long-term antiarrhythmic therapy. N Engl J Med 303:607–613, 1980.

11. IMPLANTABLE AUTOMATIC DEFIBRILLATOR NEW RESULTS IN PATIENTS

M. MIROWSKI, MORTON M. MOWER, PHILIP R. REID and LEVI WATKINS

1. INTRODUCTION

The management of ventricular fibrillation occurring outside the hospital is frequently fraught with isurmountable difficulties. Even with the continuous advances
in our understanding of the electrophysiologic and pathologic mechanisms underlying cardiac electrical activity, the delivery of a sufficiently strong electrical discharge
to the fibrillating heart is the only reliable method to terminate the lethal arrhythmia. The effectiveness of this maneuver, however, is totally dependent upon the
prompt availability of specialized personnel and equipment. In spite of the increasing availability and the improved yield of the prehospital emergency care systems
[1–3], these prereqisites for a successful defibrillation can only rarely be met outside
a medical facility. Thus, the present toll of sudden arrhythmic death remains
excessively high, reaching the awesome figure of some 450 000 victims annually in
the United States alone [4].

The problem of sudden death from ventricular fibrillation has been described as
the major challenge facing contemporary cardiology [5]. While primary prevention
through identification, reduction, and eventually elimination of the risk factors
responsible for ischemic heart disease is the ideal solution, in clinical practice
antiarrhythmic agents are the present mainstay of therapy. Unfortunately, in spite
of the continuing addition of new experimental drugs to our armamentarium [6], no
satisfactory long-term medications are yet available. There are no data, moreover,
to indicate that long-term suppressive therapy alters the occurrence of subsequent
sudden cardiac death [7]. The surgical feasibility of techniques aimed at the excision of arrhythmogenic foci from the heart has also been demonstrated and these
methods are eing ncresingly used with promise in some patients whose malignant
ventricular arrhythmias are refractory to medical therapy [8–10].

2. A NEW APPROACH – THE AUTOMATIC IMPLANTABLE DEFIBRILLATOR

The multifaceted strategy for dealing with life-threatening arrhythmias occurrng
outside the hospital has recently been complemented by the development of a
clinically applicable automatic implantable defibrillator [11–13]. This electronic
device has been designed to monitor cardiac rhythm continuously, to recognize

Adgey, AAJ (ed): Acute phase of ischemic heart disease and myocardial infarction.
© *1982, Martinus Nijhoff, The Hague, Boston, London. ISBN-13: 978-94-009-7581-1*

184

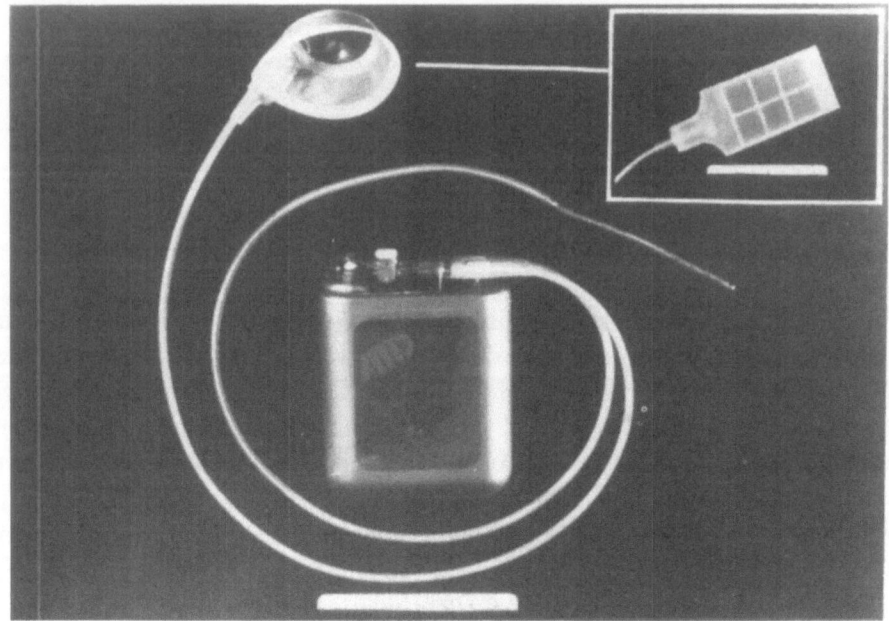

Figure 1. Automatic implantable defibrillator with its two defibrillating electrodes. The insert in the upper right corner shows the patch electrode presently preferred to the cup electrode used earlier in the study.

ventricular fibrillation, and ventricular tachycardias and then to deliver corrective defibrillatory discharges when indicated. The main objective of this approach is to protect patients at a particularly high risk of sudden arrhythmic death whenever and wherever they are struck by the lethal arrhythmia. While the monitoring, diagnostic and therapeutic capabilities of an automatic implantable defibrillator can also be provided by a coronary care unit, this device has the unique advantage of being permanently available to the patient at risk, without the need for medical assistance or additional equipment. Conceptually, the automatic implantable defibrillator can be regarded as similar to an implantable demand pacemaker, except that ventricular tachyarrhythmias rather than asystole are sensed and the delivered pulses have defibrillating characteristics.

2.1. Early experimental studies

The idea that the bulky conventional defibrillator could not only be miniaturized and implanted but also be endowed with capabilities that are now found only in specialized hospital facilities [14, 15] was received initially with skepticism. Yet, after a decade of research, these objectives have been fully achieved. Implementation of the automatic implantable defibrillator concept required, in addition to removal of conceptual obstacles, the creation of a new technology and solution of an array of engineering, electrophysiological, and clinical problems. The key to miniaturization lay in the realization that a relatively low power output is needed for internal defibrillation. Our initial research thus centered on designing electrode systems capable of defibrillating closed-chest subjects with only a small fraction of the energy needed for transthoracic defibrillation. This was achieved by developing a catheter defibrillation technique which was shown to be capable of restoring normal rhythm with pulses of some 5–20 J, while hundreds of Joules are usually required using external paddles [14, 16–19].

The first laboratory prototype of the automatic defibrillator was built and successfully tested by our group in 1969 [14]. This prototype was soon followed by more advanced models [17, 20–23] characterized by greater miniaturization, progressive refinement of the electrode and sensing systems, increased safety, and higher reliability. As a result of this effort, the size, weight, structural characteristics, and funtional performance of the implantable automatic defibrillator have reached a point where they now meet the stringent criteria required for a device suitable for implantation in human beings.

2.2. The clinical model

The physical appearance of the current clinical model is quite similar to some of the early pacemakers (Figure 1). The device* is hermetically sealed in a titanium case, weighs 250 g and occupies a volume of 145 cc. All materials in contact with body tissue are biocompatible. The two defibrillating electrodes are made from titanium and silicone rubber. One electrode is located on a catheter designed for pervenous placement in the superior vena cava near the right atrial junction. The second electrode is in the form of a cup or of a flexible rectangular patch which, for the purposes of ensuring stability of position and a low defibrillation threshold, is placed directly on the surface of the heart over the apex. The outside surface of this electrode is insulated to achieve enhanced current distribution.

The ability to monitor the heart for an extensive period of time and to promptly recognize ventricular fibrillation are essential attributes of an automatic defibrillator. A great number of approaches were investigated and tested, singly and in combination. The system which we finally adopted for clinical use establishes the diagnosis of ventricular fibrillation by identifying a specific characteristic of the arrhythmia rather than monitoring the various indirect parameters of cardiac activity such as arterial pressure, R waves, electrical impedance, etc. [24]. An important advantage of this detection scheme, in addition to its great reliability and low standby-power requirements, is its passive mode of failure. Such failure mode means that in case of a possible lead or other malfunction the device tends to remain passive, thus minimizing the possibility of an inappropriate defibrillating discharge.

---

* Developed and manufactured by Medrad, Inc./Intec Systems, Inc., Pittsburgh, Pa. U.S.A., under the name of AID®.

The sensor's logic is based on a continuous analysis of the probability density function of the differentiated ventricular electrical activity [24]. This function reflects the time spent by the slope of the input electrogram between two amplitude limits located, in our particular system, near zero potential. The probability density is a measure of how much time a signal spends, on the average, at different amplitude levels. In essence, ventricular fibrillation is identified by the striking absence of isoelectric potential segments. Ventricular tachycardias which satisfy the probability density criteria and which are faster than a preset cut-off rate are now also recognized by the device.

The power sources of the device are specially developed lithium batteries, characterized by high-energy density for prolonged life in a standby mode and by high peak power density to allow charging of the capacitors in about 10 s or less when required. Conservatively speaking, these batteries have a projected monitoring life of three years or a discharge capability of over 100 shocks.

Schuder's truncated exponential pulses [25] have been selected for use in the implantable defibrillator. Such pulses are simple to generate and for a given defibrillation efficacy require lower peak voltage and current than inductor-capacitor and simple capacitor discharges. In order for the device to deliver the predetermined amount of energy, the pulse duration ranges between 3 and 8 ms to compensate for the variations of the heart-electrode resistance.

Using Schuder's waveform, the device delivers defibrillatory shocks of 25 J about 15 s after onset of the dysrhythmia and can recycle as many as three times during a single episode if needed. The strength of the third and fourth shocks is increased to 35 J of energy. After the fourth shock, about 35 s of nonfibrillating rhythm are required to reset the counter and to allow a full series of pulses to be delivered again at the next episode. Under special clinical circumstances, when it has been determined that the 25 J might not be sufficient for defibrillation of an individual patient, pulse generators having energy output up to 45 J are also available.

2.3. Preclinical tests

A significant effort extending over more than three years was made in order to ensure that this first clinical version of the implantable automatic defibrillator would perform in a safe, effective and reliable manner [12]. Thus, in order to evaluate the long-term functional performance of the device, a chronic animal model was designed in which the syndrome of sudden death from ventricular fibrillation could be reproduced in active, conscious, dogs [11]. For this purpose a small, implantable, magnetically activated, alternating current generator with a right ventricular catheter was designed. By placing a magnet over the skin in the area where such a fibrillator is implanted, a 60 Hz current is produced and transmitted to the heart. The so induced ventricular fibrillation leads to circulatory arrest and syncope within seconds. In contrast, however, to what happens to patients stricken by this lethal arrhythmia, the animals with chronically implanted defibrillators are automatically resuscitated [11, 12].

The anatomic effects on the heart of chronic electrode implantation and of defibrillatory discharges were studied in the dog for up to 11 months after implantation and found to be minimal. In the absence of infectious complications only mild apical pericardial and epicardial fibrosis were found. Multiple shocks produced no signs of macro- or microscopic myocardial injury [12]. The preclinical testing program also included the analysis of the long-term bench performance of the defibrillator and of the effects on it of exposure to various physical stresses such as vacuum, pressure, temperature cycling, mechanical vibrations and shocks, and to the presence of electromagnetic interference signals. Despite the fact that many of the test conditions exceeded the standards required of implantable pacemakers, the results were satisfactory and the few failure modes detected were analyzed and corrected. In addition, the Applied Physics Laboratory of The Johns Hopkins University made an independent evaluation of the device which included basic device design, provocative challenges to the sensing system, analysis of components, manufacturing and quality control procedures, and of the preclinical test results. On the basis of this information the device was found suitable for use in a clinical setting [12].

2.4. In vivo evaluation of the implanted defibrillator

The question how to determine the operational readiness and reliability of a clinical device after its permanent implantation also required an answer. Such information is particularly important because the implanted unit is required to remain reliable for very long periods of time despite its apparent quiescence. The problem was solved by designing a method allowing for frequent non-invasive evaluation of defibrillator function in vivo [26]. The procedure involves triggering of a capacitor charging cycle with a magnet and then delivering the charge into a built-in test-load resistor. A specially developed defibrillator analyzer* measures the charging time by means of an electromagnetic transducer (Figure 2). Progressive increases in this time, normally 10 s or less, reflect battery depletion, whereas failure to initiate the cycle indicates abnormal operation of the device. The simplicity and the non-traumatic nature of this procedure markedly enhance the clinical applicability of the automatic defibrillator.

2.5. Patient selection

A clinical evaluation study of the automatic defibrillator began in February 1980, at The Johns Hopkins Hospital and has recently been expanded to the Stanford University Hospital as well. The patient entry criteria have been described pre-

---

* Developed and manufactured by Medrad, Ic./Intec Systems, Inc., Pittsburgh, Pa., U.S.A., under the name AIDCHECK™.

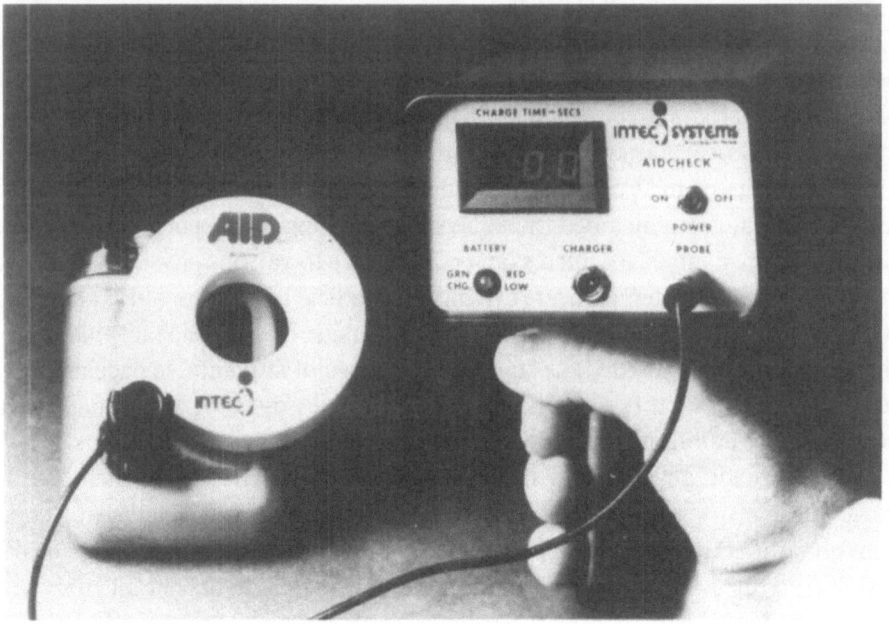

Figure 2. The defibrillator analyzer. A magnet and an electromagnetic transducer are placed over the automatic defibrillator pulse generator. For further details see text.

viously [13, 27, 28]. The prospective candidates for implantation must have survived at least two episodes of cardiac arrest outside the setting of acute myocardial infarction, with ventricular fibrillation or sinusoidal ventricular tachycardia documented electrocardiographically at least once. It was required that one such episode must have occurred despite treatment with a medication suppressing all complex ventricular arrhythmias present or, failing that, despite treatment with two anti-arrhythmic agents given simultaneously and resulting in satisfactory blood levels. Patients were excluded if they had other chronic or acute illness, were on drugs other than antiarrhythmics known to influence electrical activity of the heart, or had psychological disabilities. The extremely poor prognosis of patients fulfilling these stringent criteria is exemplified by the fact that nine patients identified as potential candidates for implantations of the automatic defibrillator died before they could be transferred to The Johns Hopkins Hospital; in some instances, they died despite being observed in a closely monitored hospital environment.

Although a total of twenty-four patients have undergone implantation of the automatic defibrillator through June 1981, detailed results are presented only for the initial sixteen patients operated on at The Johns Hopkins Hospital between February 1980, and March 1981 [28]. There were twelve men and four women whose ages at the time of surgery ranged from 16 to 74 (mean: 51 years). Coronary artery disease was the underlying heart lesion in eleven patients, non-ischemic cardio-

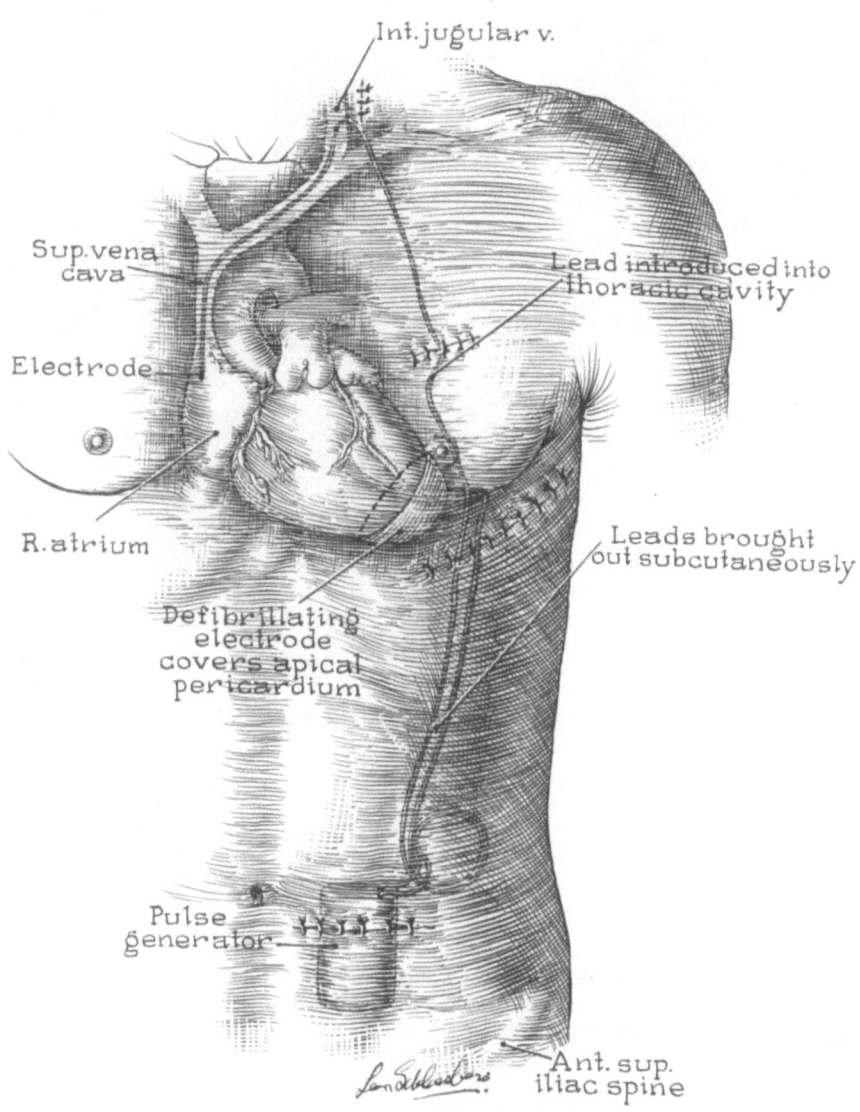

Figure 3. Schematic representation of the automatic defibrillator implantation: the lateral thoracotomy approach. The superior vena cava electrode catheter is introduced into the left internal jugular vein and positioned under fluoroscopy. The thorax is entered via the fifth intercostal space, and the apical electrode sutured to the pericardium over the cardiac apex. Both electrode leads are passed under the left costal margin. After proper insertion of the leads into the receptacle of the pulse generator, the unit is placed in the subcutaneous abdominal pocket.

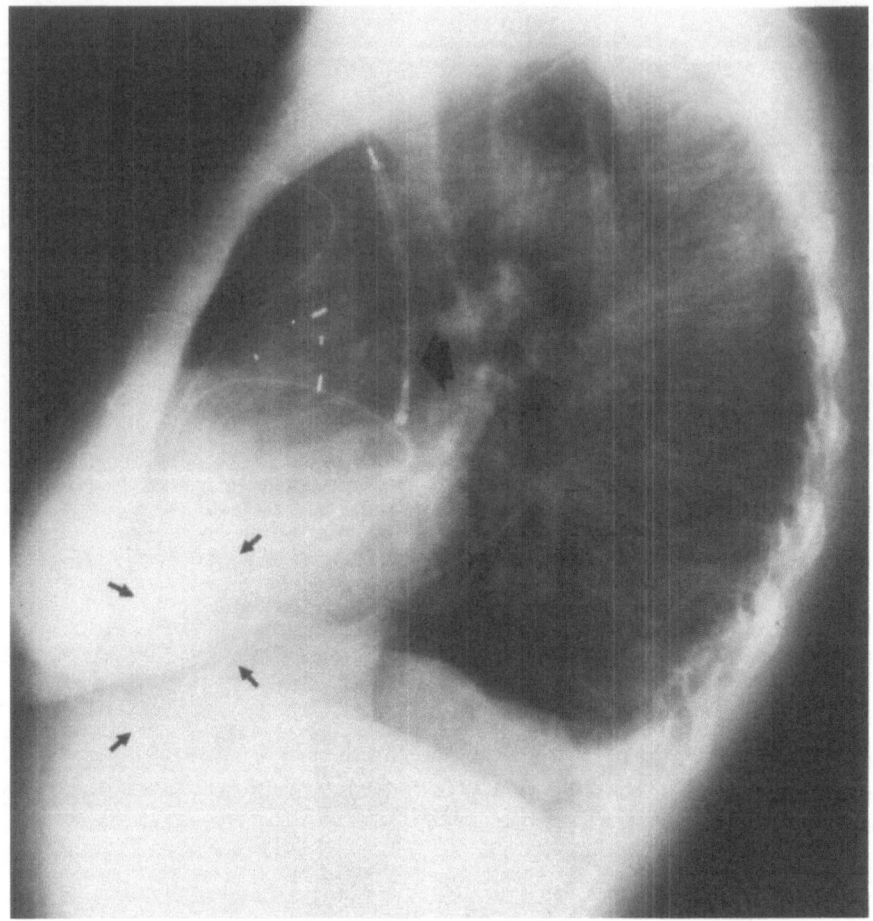

Figure 4. Lateral chest X-ray of a patient following implantation of the automatic defibrillator. The large arrow points towards the superior vena cava catheter electrode. The four small arrows point toward the radiopaque frame of the apical patch electrode.

myopathy in five: congestive in two patients, hypertrophic in two, and sarcoid in one patient. Three patients had previous coronary bypass surgery, one an aneurysmectomy, one a mitral valve prosthesis, one a septal myectomy, and three had pacemakers implanted. All but one of these patients had very poor left ventricular function. The average follow-up was six months, the longest being fourteen months.

2.6. *Implantation procedures*

A left thoracotomy was the initial surgical technique used [13]. This approach (Figure 3) is still performed in most patients who have had chest surgery in the past so as to avoid dissection at the previously operated site. Subsequently, median sternotomy has been preferred for patients without previous thoracotomy. This procedure resulted in a significant shortening and simplification of the implantation and in a decrease of the postoperative discomfort [29]. More recently, a subxiphoidal technique has been introduced [30], obviating entirely the need for a thoracotomy, thus representing a significant technical and clinical advance.

The left lateral thoracotomy technique was used in seven patients and median sternotomy in nine. The apical patch was found preferable to the cup electrode and has been implanted in all but one patient (Figure 4). Associated surgical procedures were frequently performed along with the implantation, including coronary bypass grafts (three patients), endocardial resection (one), aneurysmectomy and endocardial resection (two), and coronary bypass grafting with mitral valve replacement (one); a total of seven patients (44%) underwent these additional procedures. Also, three patients received permanent demand pacemakers. Replacement of the initially implanted pulse generators with units incorporating improved circuitry was performed in six patients. There has been no operative or hospital mortality and the postoperative morbidity was unremarkable; in general, the device has been well tolerated by the implantees. Three additional patients have undergone implantation of defibrillating electrodes during a thoracotomy for unrelated conditions and are not yet included in this series. Pulse generators may yet be implanted at a later date in these patients if indicated.

2.7. Early clinical results

Twenty-five episodes of malignant arrhythmias wich activated the automatic defibrillator were documented in the hospital following implantation; eight episodes occurred spontaneously, and seventeen were induced during electrophysiological studies. All spontaneous and fourteen of the seventeen induced arrhythmias were reverted to sinus rhythm with a single 25 J pulse (Figures 5 and 6). Slow rate and nonsinusoidal tachycardias not expected to be recognized and corrected by the device were not included in this analysis.

In three instances the induced arrhythmias, although properly identified, were not reverted by the initial discharge and the devices did not recycle promptly as expected; in one of these episodes a ventricular tachycardia accelerated into flutter-fibrillation. External countershock was used to terminate the three episodes. The delay in recycling was found to be due to transient polarization of the electrode caused by the defibrillatory discharge leading to attenuation of the input signal. Design modifications to eliminate this effect were implemented and in one subsequent case when the initial discharge and an ensuing external countershock were both ineffective, the implanted unit did recycle as programmed, delivering a second pulse which restored normal rhythm.

With only the one above-described exception, the automatic discharges were not associated with ventricular irritability, bradyarrhythmias, or asystole. Correction of the malignant rhythms with restoration of normal circulation was usually unevent-

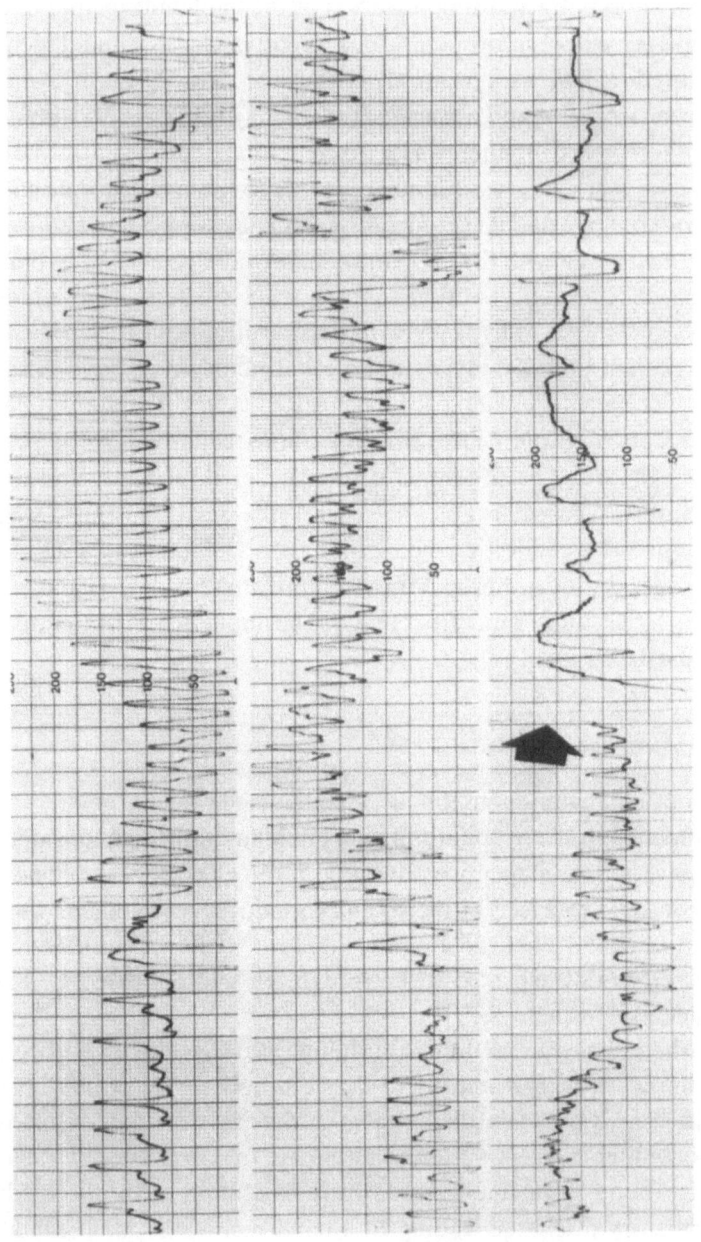

Figure 5. Record of a patient who developed atrial flutter with rapid and irregular ventricular response of 28 min duration during which the implanted automatic defibrillator remained quiescent. The last few beats of this rhythm are seen in the left part of the upper strip. Two spontaneous premature ventricular contractions then induced ventricular flutter-fibrillation and 23 s later (arrow) the malignant arrhythmia is automatically terminated by a single 25 J discharge. The strips are continuous.

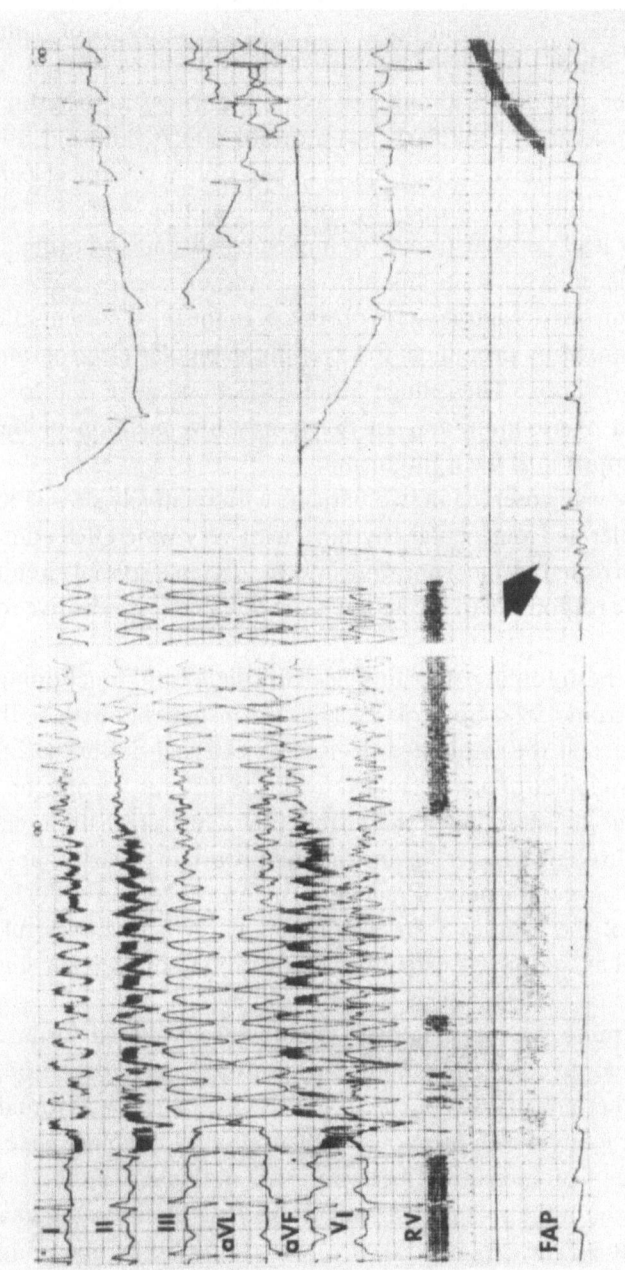

Figure 6. Left panel: initiation of ventricular flutter-fibrillation by a burst of rapid ventricular pacing. Right panel (arrow): automatic reversion of the arrhythmia to normal sinus rhythm by the implanted defibrillator. I, II, III, aVL, aVF, and V₁ are standard ECG leads. RV, right, ventricular electrogram; FAP, femoral artery pressure.

ful and virtually instantaneous. On many occasions the defibrillatory pulses were delivered to still conscious patients without producing undue discomfort or pain, confirming our initial experience [13].

In three patients a number of spurious discharges occurred during sinus rhythm. The discharges were well tolerated, produced no untoward effects, and did not induce arrhythmias. In two cases the cause was a poor connection in the apical lead producing artefacts which fulfilled the probability density function criteria. Appropriate improvements in lead construction were implemented and the original pulse generators were replaced with units insensitive to the interfering signals; subsequently, no further spurious discharges were observed. In the third patient, the false-positive pulses were caused by prominent P waves in the bipolar electrogram which satisfied the sensing criteria. These huge atrial deflections were due to a combination of right atrial overloading and an excessively low position of the catheter electrode which slipped into the right atrium.

Miscounting of heart rate was observed in two patients with relatively slow (130 and 171 beats/min), well-tolerated ventricular rhythms, with very wide QRS complexes. The problem was corrected by incorporating into the design a special circuit which made the device more responsive to the actual heart rate and less sensitive to QRS morphology changes.

No interference between the automatic implantable defibrillator and functioning demand pacemakers (Medtronic 5894 Spectrax) was noted in patients with both devices implanted. The effect of the implanted devices on external defibrillation is less clearly defined. Although supportive clinical evidence did not become apparent, laboratory tests suggested shunting of the current flow when a transthoracic countershock is delivered through paddles having an inappropriate polarity, possibly decreasing the effectiveness of the pulse. Practically, such an effect can easily be eliminated by the reversal of the paddles if an external discharge is unsuccessful. Design modifications aimed at completely excluding the possibility of such current shunting are being developed.

After nearly a hundred pulse generator implant-months accumulated to date there was no evidence of random component failure, premature battery depletion, malfunctioning capacitors, hermeticity loss or case fracture. One patient was found to have a permanent lead fracture which prompted explantation of the pulse generator. No thrombo-embolic phenomena have been observed in this series.

There were three late deaths in the group: two patients died in pulmonary edema and one was found in asystole. The explanted devices were found to be operating properly and the autopsy did not disclose myocardial damage which could be attributed to the automatic implantable defibrillator.

2.8. Conversion of out-of-hospital life-threatening arrhythmias

A number of episodes strongly suggestive of automatic termination of malignant arrhythmias outside the hospital have been described by the implantees and their relatives. Unfortunately, no graphic documentation of these out-of-hospital re-suscitations is available. Recently, however, a patient who developed severe palpitations and hypotension managed to reach a hospital emergency room where an electrocardiogram recorded showed automatic termination of a 187 beats/min ventricular tachycardia by the device [31].

3. CONCLUSIONS

These early clinical data warrant a number of conclusions. The automatic implantable defibrillator has been shown capable of reliably monitoring cardiac electrical activity for a prolonged period of time, recognizing ventricular fibrillation along with some ventricular tachycardias and delivering effective treatment. The safety record in this initial pilot study is satisfactory and all the problems which became apparent were identified and corrected. The overall results are most encouraging.

Although its ultimate role in the prevention of sudden arrhythmic deaths has yet to be determined, this new therapeutic modality represents a new and promising approach for patients who are at a particularly high risk of developing potentially lethal ventricular arrhythmias and in whom the available medical and surgical therapy is ineffective.

ACKNOWLEDGEMENTS

This study was supported in part by Grant P-50 HL 17655-07 from the National Heart, Lung, and Blood Institute, National Institute of Health.

REFERENCES

1. Pantridge JF, Geddes JS: A mobile intensive care unit in the management of myocardial infarction. Lancet 2:271–273, 1967.
2. Pantridge JF, Adgey AAJ, Geddes JS, Webb SW: The Acute Coronary Attack. pp. 104–116. New York: Grune and Stratton, 1975.
3. Cobb LA, Werner JA, Trobaugh GB: Sudden cardiac death. I and II. Mod Concepts Cardiovasc Dis 49:31, 37, 1980.
4. Lown B: Cardiovascular collapse and sudden cardiac death. In: Heart Disease (Braunwald E, ed.) p. 778. Philadelphia: WB Saunders, 1980.
5. Lown B: Sudden cardiac death: the major challenge confronting contemporary cardiology. Am J Cardiol 43:313–328, 1979.
6. Zipes DP, Troup PJ: New antiarrhythmic agents: amiodarone, aprindine, disopyramide, ethmozin, mexiletine, tocainide, verapamil. Am J Cardiol 41:1005–1024, 1978.
7. Winkle RA: Ambulatory electrocardiography and the diagnosis, evaluation and treatment of chronic ventricular arrhythmias. Prog Cardiovasc Dis 23:99–128, 1980.
8. Guiraudon G, Fontaine F, Frank R, Escande G, Etievent P, Cabrol C: Encircling endocardial

ventriculotomy: a new surgical treatment for life-threatening ventricular tachycardias resistant to medical treatment following myocardial infarction. Ann Thorac Surg 26:438–444, 1978.

9. Josephson MD, Harken AH, Horowitz LN: Endocardial excision: a new surgical technique for the treatment of recurrent ventricular tachycardia. Circulation 60:1430–1439, 1979.

10. Gallagher JJ, Cox JL: Status of surgery for ventricular arrhythmias. Circulation 60:1440–1442, 1979.

11. Mirowski M, Mower MM, Langer A, Heilman MS, Schreibman J: A chronically implanted system for automatic defibrillation in active conscious dogs. Experimental model for treatment of sudden death from ventricular fibrillation. Circulation 58:90–94, 1978.

12. Mirowski M, Mower MM, Bhagavan BS, Langer A, Kolenik SA, Fischell RE, Heilman MS: Chronic animal and bench testing of the implantable automatic defibrillator. In: Proceedings of the VIth World Symposium on Cardiac Pacing (Meere C, ed.) Chap. 27. Montreal, Canada, PACESYMP, 1980.

13. Mirowski M, Reid PR, Mower MM, Watkins L, Gott VL, Schaule JF, Langer A, Heilman MS, Kolenik SA, Fischell RE, Weisfeldt ML: Termination of malignant ventricular arrhythmias with an implanted automatic defibrillator. N Engl J Med 303:322–324, 1980.

14. Mirowski M, Mower MM, Staewen WS, Tabatznik B, Mendeloff AI: Standby automatic defibrillator: an approach to prevention of sudden coronary death. Arch Intern Med 126:158–161, 1970.

15. Schuder JC, Stoeckle H, Gold JH, West JA, Keskar PY: Experimental ventricular defibrillation with an automatic and completely implanted system. Trans Am Soc Artif Int Organs 16:207–212, 1970.

16. Mirowski M, Mower MM, Staewen WS, Denniston RH, Tabatznik B, Mendeloff AI: Ventricular defibrillation through a single intravascular catheter electrode system. Clin Res 19:328, 1971. (Abstract.)

17. Mirowski M, Mower MM, Staewen WS, Denniston RH, Mendeloff AI: The development of the transvenous automatic defibrillator. Arch Intern Med 129:773–779, 1972.

18. Mirowski M, Mower MM, Gott VL, Brawley RK: Feasibility and effectiveness of low-energy catheter defibrillation in man. Circulation 47:79–85, 1973.

19. Heilman MS, Langer A, Mower MM, Mirowski M: Analysis of four implantable electrode systems for automatic defibrillator. Circulation 52 (Suppl II):II-194, 1975. (Abstract.)

20. Mirowski M, Mower MM, Langer A, Heilman MS: Implanted defibrillators: In: Proceedings of the Cardiac Defibrillation Conference, Purdue University, West Lafayette, 1975, p. 93.

21. Mirowski M, Mower MM, Langer A, Heilman MS: Miniaturized implantable automatic defibrillator for prevention of sudden death from ventricular fibrillation. In: Proceedings, International Symposium on Cardiac Pacing, Tokyo, Japan (Watanabe Y, ed.) p. 103. Amsterdam: Excerpta Medica, 1976.

22. Mirowski M, Mower MM, Bhagavan BS, Langer A, Heilman MS, Schreibman J: The automatic implantable defibrillator: toward the development of the first clinical model. In: Proceedings of the Symposium On Management of Ventricular Tachycardia: Role of Mexiletine. p. 655. Amsterdam: Excerpta Medica, 1978.

23. Mirowski M, Mower MM, Langer A, Heilman MS: The automatic implantable defibrillator: A new avenue. In: Sudden Death (Kulbertus HE, Wellens HJJ, eds.) p. 335. The Hague: Martinus Nijhoff, 1979.

24. Langer A, Heilman MS, Mower MM, Mirowski M: Considerations in the development of the automatic implantable defibrillator. Med Instrum 10:163–167, 1976.

25. Schuder JC, Rahmoeller GA, Stoeckle H: Transthoracic ventricular defibrillation with triangular and trapezoidal waveforms. Circ Res 19:689–694, 1966.

26. Langer A, Heilman MS, Mower MM, Mirowski M: Functional analysis of the automatic implantable defibrillator in vivo. Med Instrum 12:55, 1978. (Abstract).

27. Mirowski M, Mower MM, Reid PR: The automatic implantable defibrillator. Am Heart J 100: 1089–1092, 1980.

28. Mirowski M, Reid PR, Watkins L, Weisfeldt ML, Mower MM: Clinical treatment of life-threatening ventricular tachyarrhythmias with the automatic implantable defibrillator. Am Heart J 100:265–270, 1981.

29. Watkins L, Mirowski M, Mower MM, Reid PR, Griffith LSC, Vlay SC, Weisfeldt ML, Gott VL: Automatic defibrillation in man: the initial surgical experience. J Thorac Cardiovasc Surg. 82:492–500, 1981.
30. Watkins L, Mirowski M, Mower MM, Reid PR, Freund P, Thomas A, Weisfeldt ML, Gott VL: Implantation of the automatic defibrillator: the sub-xiphoid approach. Ann Thorac Surg (In press).
31. Mirowski M, Reid PR, Mower MM, Watkins L: Successful conversion of out-of-hospital life-threatening arrhythmias with the implanted automatic defibrillator. Am Heart J 103:147–148, 1982.

200